2011   Joe & Shirley Martin

D0970926

Empowering the Patient

How to reduce the cost of healthcare *and* improve its quality

Glen E. Miller, M.D.

First published by Dog Ear Publishing
4010 West 86th Street, Suite H
Indianapolis, IN 46268
www.dogearpublishing.net

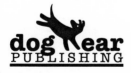

ISBN: 978-160844-156-3

This book is printed on acid-free paper.

Printed in the United States of America

CONTENTS

PART III:
Further Exploration of Healthcare Issues

INTRODUCTION

John, a writer and teacher, knows how to communicate—yet when he goes to the doctor he inexplicably clams up. Recently, John went to his doctor for vaguely felt stomach soreness. After the exam, John's doctor made an appointment for John to see a stomach specialist. The specialist explained that he would be looking at John's stomach with a light under mild anesthesia. When I asked John why they were doing the exam, he said, "I don't know why. I don't know what they suspect or what they're looking for. I get so frustrated with myself that, when I'm with the doctor, I can't think of a single question to ask."

You may have had an experience like John's where you "clammed up" in the doctor's office. It could be that you feel that the doctor has all the information—and the power that goes with that. You don't know what questions to ask or even if you have the *right* to ask questions.

This book will help you to actively participate *with* your doctor in your healthcare decisions. By doing so you will gain a sense of control, lower the cost, and improve the quality of your healthcare. The U.S. healthcare system is on life support; stated differently, it is at a crossroads. You can be part of the solution to this growing crisis.

U.S. healthcare system is failing

At the end of 2008 one-third of all U.S. residents owed money on medical bills. Forty-seven million people were without health insurance, and additional millions were (and are) one serious illness or injury away from bankruptcy. Healthcare costs are the major factor in more than 60% of personal bankruptcies. Eighteen thousand uninsured people die each year because they lack access to healthcare. Each year there are 94,000 preventable deaths in our nation's hospitals. Among all nations of the world, the powerful U.S.A. is 42nd in life expectancy, 37th in infant mortality rate, and 24th in average years of life free of disability.

The healthcare system in this country is failing—and yet, the *cost* of healthcare per person per year in the United States is more than twice as high as in other developed countries.

There is general agreement from diverse sources that cost is *the* major problem in the U.S. system of healthcare. There are many reasons that the U.S. per capita costs are much higher that other developed countries. Waste, inefficiencies in healthcare delivery, high administrative costs (including profits for insurance companies), the need for doctors to protect themselves from lawsuits, and the high demand for medical services all play a part.

'Regardless of the coming measures to reform the healthcare system at the national level, lowering costs will be essential to the success of providing affordable healthcare to all.'

At the time of this writing, politicians and healthcare industry leaders are struggling to find solutions to the healthcare crisis. In the effort to provide affordable, quality healthcare for all U.S. citizens, it is absolutely imperative that ways are found to rein in costs. *Regardless of the coming measures to reform the healthcare system at the national level, lowering costs will be essential to the success of providing affordable healthcare to all.*

Empowerment

The premise of this book is that *you*, the consumer of healthcare, can have a major impact on the cost of healthcare. In the process of lowering costs, you can actually *improve* the quality of care. This is a win/win situation.

The doctor-patient relationship is going through dramatic changes. The doctor as the all-knowing, parent-like figure and the patient as the unknowing, child-like figure are rapidly passing from the scene. Many patients are now much better educated and can access vast, diverse sources of medical information with a few clicks on the computer. And the local public library remains a gold mine of medical information.

The change, then, is from a parent-child relationship to a collaborative relationship between adults. In this arrangement, the doctor/provider is saying to the patient/consumer, *Your health is **your** responsibility. What you want, I want: to help you realize the best health possible for you to live up to your potential. I am here as a source of information and as a guide for you to achieve that.*

In this collaborative relationship the patient is saying to the doctor, *I accept that my health is my responsibility. As we cooperate in this effort, I ask you to recognize and honor my thoughts and feelings about how we achieve our common goal of maximizing my health. You have the necessary knowledge and judgment for that. I will have questions, as well as some answers from my own research, and I trust that our communication can be open and mutually respectful.*

In Haiti people say *"Si Dïeu vle"* and slap the backs of their hands in a despairing gesture as a way of saying events are out of our control; it's only as God wishes. In Egypt the corresponding expression is *"Enshallah."* When illness strikes, we may feel like victims without any control. This book will point the way to more involvement and sense of control with regard to your own healthcare.

More healthcare is not necessarily better healthcare

We might assume that more intensive medical care is better medical care. In other words, if one lab test or scan is good, two or three must be great! We may think that the doctors who are aggressive in ordering tests and surgery are better doctors. Well, as the old song says, it ain't necessarily so.

A recent *New York Times* editorial stated that:

> Some respected analysts suggest that as much as 30 percent of all health care spending in this country— some $700 billion a year—may be wasted on tests and treatments that *do not improve the health* [emphasis added] of the recipients. If even half that money could be recaptured, the amount saved would be more than enough to finance health care reforms.[1]

Atul Gawande, writing in *The New Yorker,*[2] compared the quality and cost of healthcare in the neighboring cities of McAllen and El Paso, Texas, with demographically similar populations. He noted a huge difference in the cost of healthcare per patient between the two cities and wanted to find out why. His findings do not reflect well on the doctors in McAllen. After extensive interviews with physicians, hospital administrators and public health officials, Gawande concluded that healthcare costs in McAllen are higher because

the McAllen doctors have a tendency to base medical decisions on the *financial return to the doctor*. In other places,
such as the Mayo Clinic in Rochester, Minnesota, he noted
that doctors on *salaries* worked more in teams *for the benefit
of the patient*—and *with significant cost savings*.

Dr. Elliott Fisher with others[3] in several studies involving
thousands of patients compared the level of the intensity of
healthcare to the *quality* of that healthcare and to patients'
perception of quality of their healthcare. The researchers concluded that more is *not* better: In short, more healthcare did
not improve the quality of care *nor* did it improve the
patients' perception of the quality of care they were receiving.
These findings held true for both elderly Medicare patients
and those ages 19–69.

How this book can help

Each of first 10 chapters of *Empowering the Patient* starts
with a dilemma and includes one or more actual descriptions
of patient-doctor encounters. These scenarios were discussed
with two focus groups. One group, acting as *consumers* of
healthcare, included 10 people who work for a large retirement center/nursing home. The center permitted these people
to meet on company time in eight one-hour sessions. Each
week they read a scenario and responded to specific questions. Their answers were compiled and checked back with
them at the following session.

The second focus group consisted of four doctors, three nurse
practitioners, a school nurse, two hospital-based nurses, and a
hospital chaplain. This *provider* group, which met over a period
of seven weeks, discussed the same stories of doctor-patient
encounters, as well as the responses of the consumer group.

They responded to a separate set of questions. These two focus groups, along with my personal experiences during nearly three decades of medical practice, form the basis for the sections titled *The patient's point of view, The doctor's point of view* and practical *What you can do* lists at the end of each chapter.

'I hope this introduction to one doctor will help individuals come to know their doctors as fellow human beings.'

Part II of the book is autobiographical. As I worked with the focus group of "patients," several people said they had difficulty imagining any kind of open and free discussion with their doctor. It's as if they don't see doctors as members of the human race. These essays are from my personal experience. I hope this introduction to one doctor will help individuals come to know their doctors as fellow human beings. For example, one chapter talks about the need to balance the science of medicine with compassion and how I learned that it's permissible (even helpful) for a doctor to sometimes show feeling in patient encounters. Another chapter profiles people I have known (like Mother Teresa in India) who inspired me with their dedication to justice and to care for others.

The third section is a more in-depth look at some of the issues raised in the opening chapters, such as:
- Why the cost of healthcare is so high
- How to choose a primary care physician (PCP)—or family doctor
- The place of prescription drugs in our society

This section also includes a chapter on how the Amish deal with healthcare costs in view of the fact that their religious beliefs prohibit them from buying insurance.

Your part in the healthcare crisis—and the healthcare solution

Your active participation in your own healthcare decisions *can* make a difference. Through a collaborative relationship with your doctor, you can bring down the cost of healthcare *and* improve the quality of care.

Will these measures alone solve the healthcare crisis? Certainly not. Can a single individual make a difference? Yes, along with many individuals working together. Not too long ago, as the price of gasoline rose to $4 a gallon, people found ways to conserve gas by driving slower, carpooling, combining errands, biking around town, buying/and driving more fuel-efficient vehicles and taking fewer vacations. Nationwide, there was nearly a 10% reduction in the amount of gas used. A similar, broadly based effort to reduce the costs of healthcare can have similar results.

You need no longer be a powerless, passive recipient of healthcare, but you can become an active participant, doing your part to move past the crisis and bring quality, affordable healthcare to everyone in this country. This is empowerment.

In summary, this book is designed to empower patients to save money *and* improve the quality of healthcare by (1) relating to their primary care physician in new ways of collaboration, (2) telling stories of patient-doctor encounters to educate patients where change is possible and (3) creating practical "What you can do" lists that will decrease costs without sacrificing the quality of care.

Together we can do this.

Dr. Glen E. Miller

August 2009

PART I

Doctor-Patient Encounters

CHAPTER ONE

Cost of Medicines:
You *Can* Do Something About It

The dilemma

You go to a doctor with a specific problem. After your consultation, the doctor tells you that you need a certain many-syllable medicine. You trust the doctor to know what to prescribe, but the cost of the pills is astronomical. What can you do?

An office visit—Part 1

I went to see my cardiologist (yes, even doctors go to the doctor sometimes). The cardiologist said I needed an antibiotic for the cough I had for three weeks. He asked me if I had drug insurance. When I replied that I did not, he said, "Well, that rules out the medicine I was going to give you because it costs $550 for a 10-day supply." He decided to give me a medicine that costs "only" $110. When I asked about the less expensive medicine, he said, "Actually, the $550 antibiotic is a repackaging of an older form of the same medicine. The pharmaceutical companies do that to extend the patent so they can charge a higher price." He assured me that the older medicine was just as effective as its newer, more expensive, form.

The older antibiotic cleared up my cough. I decided to question my doctor when I returned (see "An office visit—Part 2" below); I wanted to find out why he would even want to prescribe a medicine that cost five times more than the one he ended up giving me.

The patient's point of view

As consumers, advertising plays a role in fixing certain drugs in our minds (and in doctors' minds) as *the* medicine for a given condition. Some patients *want* the latest drug they learned about from an ad during a Bears-Colts football game or on the evening news. You may appreciate it when your doctor gives you a starter sample of a new drug, but you may end up paying more for filling the full prescription for the new medicine than you would have paid for a generic alternative.

Many patients assume that their doctor knows the details of their insurance policy. This may not be the case. Your doctor is probably unaware of your policy specifics, such as the amount of your co-pay and whether or not you carry any supplemental insurance, such as prescription-drug insurance.

Some people may not feel comfortable talking about money with their doctor. One woman said she did not want to be perceived as questioning her doctor's authority regarding medicine. She spoke with her pharmacist instead, asking the pharmacy to call the doctor to find out if a less expensive alternative was available.

The doctor's point of view

Most doctors are busy people, and unless you bring up the subject of cost, it may not be discussed. You should not assume that your doctor is giving you the least expensive form of the medicine. Doctors are well aware of the recently instituted "four dollars per month per drug" put forth by pharmaceutical companies and may prescribe with that in mind. (See the "What you can do ..." list at the end of this chapter for more information.) However, patients should not assume that is the case.

'You should not assume your doctor is giving you the least expensive form of medicine.'

Many doctors have stopped seeing drug representatives and accepting favors. Providers who work with mentally ill patients may continue to see drug reps because they need the samples as starter medicines. For these patients, the cost of medicines in some cases needs to include the cost of blood tests to monitor the effectiveness of those medicines.

How do doctors decide what to prescribe? According to studies, a doctor will generally remember several medicines for a given situation. Say you have a nasty cough. Your doctor will recall the drugs to treat bronchitis, think about each drug's effectiveness as applied to your case and weigh that against possible side effects. Most doctors seldom consider the *cost* of the medicine they prescribe.

Likewise, few doctors prescribe medicines because of the drug company that produces them. Drug companies are hoping that their marketing will create a fixed response in a doctor's mind. When you come into the office with knee pain due to arthritis, it may be that Advil automatically springs to your doctor's mind as the medicine of choice. Doctors tend to remember most drugs first of all by their proprietary (more expensive) names rather than their generic (less expensive) names. For instance, Zocor may more readily spring to mind for the treatment of high cholesterol than the generic name Simvastatin.

An office visit—Part 2

When I saw my cardiologist six months later, I reminded him of our previous conversation and asked, "If you felt the older, cheaper medicine would do just as well, why did you initially prescribe the newer medicine that was five times more expensive?"

The good doctor went into a rather long explanation that can best be summarized by saying he thought the newer medicine is what I would want. After I expressed my concern about the high cost of health-care in general, the cardiologist looked over the other medicines I was taking and changed one of them to its generic form. This change reduced the cost of that medicine from $1.85 to $0.59 per day—a savings of $463 per year.

Later I took advantage of the special drug company offer of $4 per month per drug and saved an additional $167 per year on this medicine for a total savings of $630 a year—or $52.50 per month.

Remember ...

Several things should now be clear. Doctors don't automatically pay attention to the cost of the medicine they prescribe, they likely won't know your insurance status and they feel the pressure of a limited amount of time with each patient. As a result, you may be given a prescription for medicine that is the most expensive when another less expensive medicine may be just as effective. You, the patient, need to *ask* about the cost of medicine so the cost automatically becomes part of the decision of which medicine is best.

What you can do to reduce the cost of prescription drugs

1. Tell your doctor that the cost of healthcare is important to you and that you want to know about the cost of tests, procedures, services and medicines.
2. Recognize that the newest medicine may not be the most effective.
3. Ask your doctor for generic drugs when available.
4. Ask your doctor for larger prescriptions that will last for a longer period of time and will result in lower cost of the medication per day.
5. Take advantage of drug companies' special offers. Check with your local pharmacy about a "$4 per month per drug" limit on prescriptions (those covered can be found online). An annual fee for a $35 card was established by many pharmaceutical companies in 2008 and renewed in 2009.
6. Check prices of medicines online. Then in light of your research, you can ask the doctor's office to fax a prescription to your pharmacy.
7. Get the larger size pill and split it in half to get the same dosage of medicine at a reduced cost per day.
8. Check *http://www.consumerreports.org/health/best-buy-drugs/index.htm* for a comparison of the efficacy and cost of drugs for specific conditions.
9. See Chapter 19, "Prescription Drugs: How to Bring Them Under Control," for more information on why medicines cost so much.

CHAPTER TWO

Eliminating Defensive Medicine: Trust Is a Key Element

The dilemma

You go to the doctor with a painful and swollen knee. You don't remember any injury to explain the symptoms. After an examination in the office, your doctor says it may be arthritis. He doesn't suggest an X-ray or blood tests. You leave with a prescription but are uneasy because you're unsure about the diagnosis and wonder if the treatment will work. What can you do?

An office visit

A pediatrician in Pennsylvania told me this story:

A mother brought her 12-year-old son to see me after the boy ("Johnny") hurt his ankle playing soccer. After examination, I explained that it looked like a typical sprain without any evidence of a broken bone. I suggested the "RICE" treatment: rest, ice, compression and elevation. I told her that in more than 95% of cases that is all that is needed. Further, I said that if Johnny did not improve in 24 hours, she should call me and I would order an X-ray to rule out bone injury.

The mother informed me that she had insurance and that she wanted an X-ray and an MRI [magnetic resonance imaging]. The cost of the office visit was $75, the X-ray $120 and the MRI $740. What started as a routine office visit costing $75 was now going to cost nearly $1,000. The X-rays and MRI showed no evidence of bone injury. The insurance paid for the X-rays and MRI.

The patient's point of view

Mother is concerned for Johnny and wants the best of care for him. The doctor says he is "95% certain" that there are no broken bones and advises the usual treatment. Johnny's mother wants the MRI because she feels that it will make sure the treatment is correct and that nothing more needs to be done. She knows that MRIs are available and used in sports medicine. The money won't come out of her pocket; her insurance will pay for it. In her view, this is why she has insurance.

In the story above, most patients would accept the advice of the doctor to wait for X-rays since the quality of care is not adversely affected by waiting for a day to see if and how the boy's symptoms subside. However, when children are younger and can't describe their symptoms, more investigation could be needed even if it adds to the cost.

'Patients feeling that they are being heard is *essential* in building trust.'

The story suggests that the mother didn't really trust the doctor and his advice to wait for X-rays. She may have had a number of reasons for her lack of trust: a sense of being rushed through the office encounter, the feeling that the doctor wasn't really listening or fully attentive, or having heard of the experience of another person in a similar situation with that doctor or even another doctor. The first issue, patients feeling that they are being heard, is *essential* in building trust. Patients report that:

a) "The doctor doesn't listen to me."
b) "When we disagree on something, he says I need counseling."
c) "I feel like I'm on a conveyor belt and have only five minutes of the doctor's time."

Patients generally agree that the actual time spent with them is less important than the feeling that they have the doctor's full attention and their concerns have been heard.

The doctor's point of view

Most doctors would agree that there was no need to order immediate X-rays for Johnny. In other situations, the issue is not as clear, such as when an athlete wants to know how long he or she must be inactive.

The pediatrician knows that in more than 95 of 100 cases of ankle sprain, the standard RICE treatment is all that is needed. He has an uneasy feeling because the boy's mother doesn't accept his suggestion that the injury can be treated conservatively. Yet he needs to address the mother's concern for more certainty, so he orders the MRI, knowing full well there's very little chance that anything will be found that requires other treatment.

Why would the pediatrician order the tests when he knows they aren't necessary for good healthcare? There may be several reasons: He might feel that he needs to keep the mom happy in order to keep her and her family as patients. Furthermore, he may justify ordering the tests knowing that if he *doesn't* order the tests, she will likely go to another doctor who *will* order the extra studies.

The doctor also may feel the need to order additional tests on the remote chance that there is a broken bone that was missed by his exam and that the delay could lead to a lawsuit. When a doctor initiates extra, largely superfluous tests, it's called defensive medicine (see next section). In the case of the sprained ankle, the pediatrician could have allayed the mother's anxieties by talking through a careful exam and then, with the mother, making a "joint" decision about the need for X-rays, which almost certainly wouldn't have been ordered if the mother had to pay for them herself.

Healthcare providers know that spending time with patients and listening carefully are vitally important. When time is limited, doctors are frustrated with the patient who comes for a routine office visit and spends time talking about non-issues like the latest weather reports and "Aunt Tillie's surgery." They suggest that patients state *all* of their concerns at the beginning of the visit so that time can be properly budgeted.

What can be done if there's a lack of trust between doctor and patient? Most doctors agree that if there's a problem of trust, it's best for the patient to discuss it openly rather than just leave. Doctors who sense a lack of trust may see it as an indication of the need to refer the patient to a specialist.

Defensive medicine

Defensive medicine is what doctors do to lessen the likelihood of getting sued. It is defined as: "A deviation from sound medical practice that is induced primarily by a threat of malpractice suits."[4] In defensive medicine the doctor proceeds with tests or treatment that do not improve the quality of care. In fact, the tests and treatment may *decrease* the quality of care. In Johnny's case, the doctor clearly thought the X-ray and MRI weren't needed. Yet he felt compelled to order these expensive tests because of the remote possibility of an injury not discovered through his clinical examination. Such a later discovery could be found to have caused delay in treatment, which in turn could lead to legal action by the patient or patient's family. In a survey[5] of doctors, 93% said they practice defensive medicine. In the same study, 92% of doctors reported ordering unnecessary tests and diagnostic procedures and making pointless referrals. That's a huge majority of physicians practicing medicine in a manner that, by definition, really doesn't improve the quality of healthcare. Why? Because *they* don't trust their patients not to sue.

Remember ...

Defensive medicine accounts for at least 3% (60 billion dollars nationally) of all healthcare costs and does virtually nothing to improve the quality of care. Most doctors and other healthcare providers feel the need to practice defensively in order prevent a lawsuit or to protect themselves in the event of court proceedings.

You, the patient, can reduce or eliminate the physician's fears of a possible lawsuit by knowing your questions before you go to the doctor and engaging in a confident and open conversation about the diagnosis and proposed treatment. Yes, *you* can do something about the costly practice of defensive medicine. When your doctor feels that you fully understand and agree with the diagnosis and treatment, it will greatly lessen his or her inclination to practice defensive medicine.

'*You* can do something about the costly practice of defensive medicine.'

Ultimately, building a trusting relationship with your doctor will lead to better healthcare. If you have insurance like Johnny's mother, you may not feel the *financial* benefits of forgoing unnecessary procedures, but developing a mutually trusting relationship with your doctor will have dividends of its own.

What you can do to build trust between you and your doctor

1. Insist on a full and understandable explanation of the plan for diagnosis, including the need for lab tests, X-rays or scans.
2. Be sure you understand how you will know if the treatment is effective:
   a) When can you expect improvement, such as decreased fever or less pain?
   b) What should you watch for?
   c) When should you call the doctor back?

3. Openly discuss any concerns you have about the recommended plan.
4. Write down or get a list of instructions from the doctor. Consider taking someone with you so you're sure to understand everything.
5. Be aware that unnecessary tests will almost certainly decrease the quality (and certainly increase the cost) of your healthcare.
6. Recognize the caregiver's limited time and go prepared with:
    a) Lists of current medications and allergies.
    b) A concise account of your present medical problem.
    c) Tell your doctor at the beginning of the visit—if you have more than one medical problem that needs attention.

CHAPTER THREE

Medical Records:
The Life You Save May Be Your Own

The dilemma

It is late at night. You are traveling 800 miles from home when you are involved in a traffic accident. The ambulance takes you to a nearby emergency room. Before you are evaluated for your injuries, the ER nurse asks about allergies to medicines. You remember that you had a severe skin rash after taking a medicine several years ago, but now you can't remember the med's name. What can you do?

An office visit

> *"James" had his usual annual physical exam with routine blood tests. Several weeks later he was feeling very tired, weak and dizzy. At the insistence of his wife, he went to see a second doctor. A blood test there showed significant anemia. James recalled the blood test he had at the time of his annual physical. He had assumed since the doctor's office didn't call, his blood test must have been normal. When he called to check on the original blood count, he was informed that there was no record of the test result.*

Anemia can be the earliest indication of a serious underlying problem, including cancer of the bowel. The lost lab result caused a delay in diagnosis and treatment and might have made it more difficult, or even impossible, to treat and cure the problem.

Another office visit

"Linda" had a superficial cancer removed from her forearm and underwent a subsequent scan to rule out the spread of the cancer. The oncology office called to say that all tests were negative. As Linda reviewed the written report a week later with her oncologist, they read the following: "The metastatic lesion is seen." That statement did not match the rest of the report, which led the oncologist to believe it must be a typo. Clearly they needed clarification. One week later, after Linda's doctor's office had made three calls to radiology, with no response, Linda wrote to her friend, a chaplain, about her frustrations. The chaplain forwarded Linda's letter to the patient advocate and director of imaging at the hospital where the tests were done. They got results the next morning. The original writer of the report was on leave in India, so the chief of radiology reviewed it and concluded that the report should have read, "No metastatic lesion is seen."

The patient's point of view

James' lab test was lost, and proper diagnosis was delayed. Although James had enough time to take the necessary steps, in other instances such negligence can have tragic consequences. Lab tests may be lost for a variety of reasons in busy doctors' offices and hospitals. When the report of Linda's scan contained the perplexing sentence, she wasn't content with the discrepancy and insisted on a clarification.

Many patients are reluctant to ask their doctor for medical records. On any visit to the medical office, they're keenly aware that their doctor and staff are very busy and should not be bothered with the seemingly trivial issue of a copy of a lab test. Many aren't even sure they have a right to ask. They may wonder, "Who do the records belong to?" Others who *have* asked for copies of medical records may have experienced reluctance on the part of the doctor's office staff to make copies. These patients also may wonder, "What is it that my doctor doesn't want me to know?"

The doctor's point of view

Doctors agree that patients have a right to copies of their medical records. They understand that many patients are more knowledgeable now and can often interpret their reports. Patients should always ask for copies of both *normal and abnormal* test results to ensure that someone has actually looked at the result. Most doctors do not routinely provide copies; patients need to ask for them.

'Patients have a right to copies of their medical records.'

When the doctor orders a test at the hospital, he or she can ask the hospital to send a copy of the report to the patient. Most medical offices provide a free copy of single page test result, but there may be a small charge for the transfer of a complete medical record.

Occasionally you may have an abnormal test result that doesn't have clinical significance. An example might be a blood sugar that is slightly elevated when the patient had not been fasting. If a patient receives an abnormal test result, most doctors prefer to personally explain the result to the patient in order to make sure the patient understands the test result. On the day of this writing, a news report said that in 7% of cases with abnormal lab results (a "shockingly high number") doctors failed to report the results to their patients.

Most doctors provide copies of lab tests and procedure results but are reluctant to give copies of their clinical notes. These are the notes in the patient's chart that include the course of the disease process, the interpretation of tests, and any social or family factor that might influence the care of the patient. The doctor's reluctance to release these notes stems from the fact that doctors may write notes to themselves about the patient; for the patient to read such notes could cause unnecessary anxiety. For example, a patient may complain of muscle weakness and occasional vague numbness. Hearing that, the doctor may write a note to watch for progressive signs of MS (multiple sclerosis), a disease that's usually very difficult to diagnose in its early stages. A note like this is written to help the doctor in the future but would likely cause the patient undue angst.

Medical records

Medical records are *essential* to good healthcare. These records include the individual's listing of past serious illnesses and operations, laboratory, X-ray and pathology reports, drug allergies, ongoing medical problems, current medications, and pertinent family medical history. In the absence of medical records, there could be critical delay in the diagnosis and treatment of a serious illness.

'In the absence of medical records, there could be a critical delay in the diagnosis and treatment of a serious illness.'

Doctors and healthcare providers have the responsibility to maintain accurate and legible medical records in an orderly manner while protecting their patients' confidentiality. The benefit of all that effort is lost if the medical records are not available to medical caregivers in the time of an emergency or ongoing care.

Remember ...

Having access to an accurate medical history at the time of an acute illness is crucial to receiving good care without delay. Patients have a right to copies of their medical records and have *every right* to ask for a copy of their records.

It is essential that any doctor taking care of you has important information like allergies, medications, past history and chronic diseases. You may *assume* that you will remember these important details in the time of an emergency. And you likely *assume* that a test result must be negative if the doctor's office didn't call. Or you *assume* that the last test result will be available when needed. Already we have three assumptions. These assumptions prove to be false thousands of times a day in this country and lead to missed diagnoses and delayed or inappropriate treatment. Rather than *assuming,* you can be *certain* that tests results will be available when needed by collecting and keeping the necessary records.

The evidence is clear:

- The number of repeat tests can be greatly reduced if the results of tests are readily available.
- There also will be a significant reduction in the need for hospitalization.
- In an emergency there will be less delay in treatment if the results of recent lab tests and a brief summary of pertinent medical history are available.
- If the patient has copies of test results, the cost of health-care will be reduced and the quality improved.

A final note: In all the discussion about changes in our healthcare system, there is rightly a great deal of emphasis on the importance of health records. The planners visualize EMR (electronic medical records) for each patient. It will take three to five years, however, to supply an EMR to all patients. In the meantime, you must take responsibility to know and maintain your own up-to-date medical record. The life you save may be your own.

What you can do about your medical records

1. Ask for copies of all results of blood tests, X-rays, scans, pathology reports and surgical reports.
2. If you don't understand a report, call your doctor's office for an explanation.
3. Get answers to the following items that a doctor will need:
   - **Patients with an acute illness** but no longstanding disease should have:
     - Record of medicines, including over-the-counter meds
     - Allergies and intolerance to meds and other sub-stances
     - Immunizations

- History of past serious illnesses and hospitalizations
- Surgeries
- Significant family history
- Name and contact information of their primary healthcare provider
- **Patients with chronic disease** should have all of the above, as well as records that include the course of their chronic disease, treatment and recent lab results.

4. Make up your own medical summary and carry a copy with you. I do. (See Chapter 20 for a sample format of a medical summary.)

5. Check out the website *Your Personal Health Information: A Guided Tour* at *http://www.myphr.com*. This is a good overview of medical records, who owns them, how they are used and suggestions about maintaining a personal copy.

CHAPTER FOUR

Chronic Disease:
In It for the Long Haul

The dilemma

Your doctor recently informed you that you have diabetes. You now must face the fact of a chronic disease—a disease that doesn't go away with treatment but is likely to be with you the rest of your life. It's depressing. What can you do?

An example

My friend Lynn recounts when he learned about his newly diagnosed diabetes.

> *When you feel bad, especially abdominally, you usually know that this too shall pass (no pun intended). But sometimes, the discomfort is different, so different that you pick up the phone and make an appointment with your family doctor. This was one of those days, not so bad to make you wish you were already dead, but bad enough to know that you need some professional advice. This didn't feel like it was going to get better by morning.*
>
> *So I picked up the phone—and an hour later entered the office of my physician. His office nurse took me*

into their little lab and pricked my index finger with a small spring-loaded knife. Then she took me back to the "cooling your heels" room where I waited to be seen by my doctor.

He came in 10 minutes later and, without asking any questions at all, announced that the blood sample showed I had diabetes, Type 2! My blood sugar was over 250 milligrams/deciliter (mg/dcl). No wonder I felt lousy; normal blood sugar should be 87 mg/dcl or so. And then my doctor pulled out a piece of paper, handed it to me, and said, "Here, follow this diet." End of visit.

What my trusty medical doctor had just handed me was the current American Diabetics Association diet recommendation for Type 2 diabetics. For a person my age and weight, the ADA recommended that I eat no more than 1600 calories per day, and 60% of that was supposed to come from carbohydrates. Great, I love bread, especially really heavy, whole-grain bread. This is going to be fun! When I got home I called my insurance provider, who promptly sent me a free blood glucose monitor kit. Free stuff to check the level of the sugar that those 960 calories of carbohydrates were producing. And check I did, about every half hour. I even bought the cable and the software that allowed me to enter my readings into my home computer and generate tables and graphs of my wondrous blood-sugar levels. On the next visit to my doctor I took the printouts of my self-monitoring, and he was duly impressed. But the numbers were still pretty high. And they went up and down like mad.

*I opened the phone book looking for more informa-
tion about diabetes treatments and monitoring to see
what I was missing, and I noticed a phone number for
a local "diabetes education service." When I called
the educator, she heard my confusion and recommended that I do a "pancreas capacity test" on
myself. This consisted of eating a measured amount of
carbohydrates, then testing my blood every half hour
for two hours to see how high it got. She recommended starting at 30 grams/meal for three meals,
then 40, then 50. Since cellular damage begins at
blood-sugar levels above 160mg/dcl, the trick was to
keep my blood sugar at or below 150.*

*There was nothing about this in the ADA material, but
it makes sense. If the aim of treating diabetes is to
keep from killing off your nerves or kidneys or eye-
sight, then keeping the blood sugar below the level
where that happens should be the main goal.*

*So I got out my normal breakfast cereal, looked at the
box to see what it contained in the way of carbohydrates and put together a breakfast that equaled 30
grams of carbohydrates. I tested my blood four times,
every half hour for the next two hours. Great! Over
three meals it never went above 150, although it did
hit 145 several times. Then I upped the carb content to
40 grams, and, oops, I got high numbers of 165, 170.
Too much.*

*Then I got out my handy-dandy calculator and did the
math on the ADA diet my doctor gave me. Let's see ...
60% of 1600 calories is 960 calories from carbohydrates, 960 calories divided by 3.5 calories/gram of*

carbohydrate equals 270 grams, 270 grams divided by three meals equals 90 grams per meal! No wonder I was seeing blood-sugar levels of 200mg/dcl and above. By following the ADA diet, I was eating three times as many carbohydrates as my pancreas—and the insulin it produced—could handle!

What is going on here? Why are my doctor and the ADA trying to kill me? I got back on my trusty computer and "Googled" Type 2 Diabetes, spending the next week reading article after article about reduced carbohydrate intake and the treatment of diabetes without medication. The conclusion I came to is that it's pretty stupid to eat the carbohydrates that raise blood-sugar levels, then buy medication to lower those blood sugars, which is what I would have to do to follow the ADA diet. Why would the ADA recommend a diet that results in taking more medication? The answer came in the mail that very month—in the form of the ADA's own magazine, Diabetes Forecast. *As I looked in vain in that magazine for an article about treating diabetes by lowering carbohydrate intake, I noticed something: Almost all the paid advertising in the magazine was either about monitoring equipment or about drugs to lower blood sugar.*

Finally, I got it. No one pays the ADA to put in an ad about eating fewer carbohydrates. No, the money is in advertising the drugs that you will need to take if you follow the ADA dietary recommendations, as well as the machines you will need to keep hourly track of your elevated blood sugar so you will know how much of that expensive medication you will need to take.

There is possibly one other reason the ADA still doesn't recommend lowering carbohydrate intake as a way of moderating your blood sugar. Can you imagine what it would take for an institution of that prestige to admit that it has been giving bad advice for the last 50 years? Why, that would be like Fidelity Investments admitting that considering expenses and fees, on average you would have been much better off investing in indexes—or stocks a chimpanzee picked—than in its highly touted mutual funds. Don't hold your breath waiting for either announcement.

The patient's point of view

In the story above, Lynn, who has no background in medical care, took it upon himself to learn what he needed to know about diabetes. (By the way, this doctor thinks he did a bang-up job of educating himself.) Diabetes is near the top of the list of chronic diseases.

A chronic disease is different from an acute illness. With an acute illness, you get sick; you get medical care, you get better, and you go home ... until the next time. But patients like Lynn with chronic diseases—diseases that don't go away—require long-term care. Many patients (and even caregivers), however, tend to treat a chronic disease as if it's an *acute* disease. They may assume that the problem will get better and delay or avoid going to see their doctor until their symptoms take a turn for the worse. For example, a patient with a burning sensation on urination goes to his doctor, gets an antibiotic and the symptoms disappear; he returns to the doctor only if the symptoms reappear. The tendency for patients with chronic diseases to show up when their symptoms appear, then disappear between episodes, has been called the "radar syndrome."

Patients intuitively know that it's better to catch a disease in its early stages, but many patients in the early stages of such illnesses as diabetes, high blood pressure or heart disease *have* no symptoms. Patients who have a family history of diabetes and high blood pressure need to get regular screening for blood sugars and blood-pressure checks. Diagnosis early in the disease may prevent life-threatening problems, such as diabetic coma, stroke or heart attack.

The doctor's point of view

Doctors agree that *responsibility and self-discipline on the part of the patient are essential to the proper control of chronic diseases.* One physician suggested a sports analogy of the doctor as the coach and the patient as the player. The doctor/coach outlines the treatment and the hoped-for outcome, but it is ultimately up to the patient/player to achieve the goals of treatment.

'Doctors agree that *responsibility and self-discipline on the part of the patient are essential to the proper control of chronic diseases.'*

Michelle, a family practitioner, has a flow sheet that lists the goals of the treatment for diabetes. At each visit she reviews with her patient the goals for blood sugar, weight, A1C (a test to monitor diabetes control) and other parameters. Together they can clearly see where they're meeting the goals of treatment and where improvement is necessary. With this approach, the doctor and patient are on the same team, sharing responsibility for meeting the goals.

Group sessions for patients with diabetes, arthritis and other chronic diseases are available in some offices and have been found to be helpful and efficient in taking care of common problems. For patients with diabetes, a doctor, nurse, dietitian and physical therapist can all meet with a group of 10 to 15 patients. In the question-and-answer period, patients learn not only from the professionals present but also from each other.

Chronic disease—the big picture

As noted at the outset of this chapter, nearly half of Americans live with at least one chronic condition. Chronic diseases account for 70% of deaths in America, more than 75% of the $2 trillion healthcare cost and about a third of the years of potential life lost before age 65. The most common chronic diseases are heart disease and strokes, diabetes, high blood pressure, cancer, arthritis and obesity.

Each of these conditions adds hugely to the total cost of healthcare. The direct cost of healthcare for persons with chronic diseases is only part of the total cost. Added to that is the indirect cost of the loss of productivity as people are sidelined due to complications of their disease. Chronic diseases generally have well-established guidelines for improving quality of life, staving off complications, preventing hospitalizations and prolonging years of active life rather than disability.

Americans are 24th in the world in disability-free life expectancy. The treatment of chronic disease to preserve function and an active life is the major factor that places 23 developed countries ahead of the U.S. in the number of years we can expect to lead an active life without disability.

Remember ...

Chronic illness requires a major attitude adjustment on the part of the patient. Your doctor cannot do it all. Become proactive and take responsibility alongside your caregiver in controlling the progression and complications of your disease. Openly discuss with your physician your need to know about your illness, understand the goals and guidelines of treatment, and accept responsibility to work toward meeting those goals.

Don't rely solely on your doctor for information. Search other sources, such as the Internet[6] and professional organizations. Lynn, in the story above, sets an excellent example.

Good long-term care and an understanding of your illness will:
- Help keep your disease under control
- Delay progression of the disease symptoms; most chronic disease symptoms get worse over time; the symptom progression can be delayed or even prevented with careful control of the disease
- Prevent the serious complications of the disease (for example, heart attack, cancer or stroke)
- Avoid unnecessary hospital stays
- Maintain your ability to be active and work productively, thereby improving your quality of life
- Decrease the cost of healthcare

What you can do about chronic disease

- Change your mindset and accept the fact that a chronic disease will require long-term (and possibly indefinite) treatment. This is an enormous, essential step.
- Establish a good working relationship with a doctor knowledgeable in the care of your chronic disease; work

together to achieve the goals of good treatment.

- Participate in screening opportunities for diabetes, high blood pressure and cancer, especially if there's a history of the condition in the family.
- Establish realistic goals of treatment with your doctor for any chronic illness, such as high blood pressure, diabetes and obesity.
- Become aware of the signs and symptoms when your chronic disease is not under control and discuss with your doctor the signs or symptoms that will alert you that you need emergency care.
- Remember that with chronic diseases, the more you know, the better you'll be able to control your disease.
- Ask your doctor for sources of information, then also search the Internet and contact professional organizations.

CHAPTER FIVE

Emergency Room:
For True Emergencies Only

Dilemma 1

Your elderly father, who had a heart attack six years ago, calls you at 8 p.m. complaining of "indigestion." You know he's taking heart medicine. You're concerned. Is this simply indigestion, or is it the start of another heart attack? Does he need emergency care?

Dilemma 2

Your talented, hard-charging daughter suffered a blow to her skull when she knocked heads with another player in a weekend soccer game. After the game, she has a knot on her forehead and a headache. How serious is her injury? Should she go to the ER?

The patient's point of view

Many individuals have access to resources that can help them decide whether they are facing an emergency (or not), whether to call an ambulance or drive to an ER. Others don't have the background or opportunities to check with medical experts to decide if their situation calls for emergency care. And some people, without too much thought, err on the side of safety and make a beeline for the nearest ER. Unfortunately, an unnecessary visit to the ER can be a very costly decision.

'An unnecessary visit to the ER can be a very costly decision.'

In cases of severe illness or injury, it will be obvious that ER care is needed. Other times the situation will be less clear. Following is a partial list of conditions when an individual clearly needs the emergency room:

- Is there bleeding or a laceration that will need stitches?
- Is the injury such that an X-ray will be required?
- Is there trouble breathing?
- Are there pronounced mental changes, such as serious confusion or loss of consciousness?
- Is there a high fever?
- Is there a recurrence of a chronic problem (asthma, for example) that required ER care before?

The doctor's point of view

Doctors recognize that there are true emergencies. They also know that at times patients run to an ER with a problem that is not truly urgent. Most doctors understand that it's sometimes difficult for patients to tell the difference.

For this reason, many primary care physicians are in a group practice or have arrangements with other doctors to provide care for problems that occur outside office hours. The on-call doctor will ask the patient to come to the office where he or she has access to the patient's records. Other PCPs have no off-hour coverage and so instruct patients to go to the local ER without knowing whether their patient is experiencing a true emergency. In the process of selecting a PCP, it's important to understand the plan for emergency care when the office is closed.

Many doctors look with favor on the use of urgent-care or walk-in clinics. These clinics provide care when the doctor's office is closed and a problem can't wait until the next office hours. These urgent-care clinics are less expensive than an emergency room and usually see patients without long waits.

> *I was at a picnic where a man was walking in a wooded area, and a small branch snapped back and hit him in the eye. He noticed pain in the eye but could still see. When the pain persisted, he called an urgent-care clinic and got an immediate appointment. The clinic doctor diagnosed the problem as a small abrasion of the eye and gave eye drops and an eye patch. The elapsed time was less than an hour and for a fraction of the cost of going to the ER of a hospital.*

Because ER doctors need to make a diagnosis in a short period of time and usually have no previous knowledge of a patient, they frequently order a "battery" of tests on admission to the ER. Also, because many malpractice lawsuits originate in the ER, doctors are understandably sensitive to this and may want to "cover" their proverbial posteriors by ordering more tests than might be warranted. A PCP who has a good relationship with a patient and knowledge of his or her past history would be able to greatly decrease both the number of tests and the costs.

PCPs can be severely hampered when their patients come to see them after a visit to the ER and there's no information available about the diagnosis and treatment they received.

Patients often don't remember the details of their emergency visit well enough to adequately inform their physician.

Emergency rooms are facing their own emergencies

Some politicians have argued that all Americans *do* have access to healthcare, since legally ERs cannot turn away a patient—unless they aren't equipped to handle a specific case or are overcrowded. Due to overuse and underpayment, the future of large numbers of ERs is in jeopardy. In the last decade, the number of *visits* to ERs has increased by 26%. During the same period, the actual number of ERs has *decreased* by 9%. As a result, most ERs are crowded, and wait times are long. If an ER is too busy, ambulances are diverted to different hospitals. Each year, more than half a million ambulances are diverted. This often costs precious time for a seriously ill patient.

While ERs cannot legally turn people away without care, there is no funding provided for the uninsured, and so a significant portion of the charges for emergency care are not paid. In a national survey, from 1996 to 2004 the percentage of ER charges for which the hospital received payment *decreased* from 57% to 42%. This has directly contributed to the closure of quite a few ERs and trauma centers. In addition, some specialists refuse to be associated with ERs due to liability issues and fear of lawsuits.

Remember ...

1. *True* emergencies belong in the emergency room, whereas routine cases don't.

2. Some communities have alternatives to the ER, such as urgent-care and walk-in clinics. Businesses, in an effort to reduce the frequency of ER visits, may have a nurse available for telephone consultation. There are also Internet services, such as Blues On Call, with a nurse available to discuss the problem (see *http://www.rollins.edu /hr/OE2005/HealthBluesOnCall.pdf*).

3. The cost of ER care is high for a number of reasons, including:
   - The need to staff for peak times when the ER is the busiest.
   - Because of the need for rapid assessments, there is a tendency to order a "battery" of tests rather than specific tests.
   - Repeat tests may be done because the results of recent tests are not readily available.
   - Those who pay must at least in part cover the current 58% of ER bills that are not paid or reimbursed.
   - Patients arriving in the ER may have delayed in seeking medical help, thereby complicating their problem and increasing the cost.
   - Because typically there isn't an ongoing relationship between patient and provider, the ER doctor will have a tendency (even a need) to practice more defensive medicine.

What you can do to avoid unnecessary ER visits and to know your alternatives

- Establish a relationship with a primary care physician.
  - Call the local hospital and ask for the doctor referral service, who in turn will tell you which doctors in the area are accepting new patients.
  - Ask what arrangement the doctor has for off-hours emergencies.

- Check if the doctor takes care of his or her patients when they're hospitalized or if they're referred to another hospital-based doctor. While this may not affect the quality of care, it's important for you to know, especially if you're one of nearly 150 million Americans with a chronic disease or health problem.
- Find out to which hospitals the doctor you're investigating has admitting privileges.
- Check with friends for recommendations.
- Gather the necessary records of your past medical problems and history to take to the first visit with your new doctor.

- Discuss with your doctor arrangements for emergency coverage in off hours.
- In cases of a chronic and recurrent problem, develop a clear concept with him or her of what constitutes an emergency.
- Have a summary copy of your medical records available to hand to ER attendants.
- Learn procedures to assess the severity of an acute illness or injury.
- Learn other places to call to discuss the severity of a problem with a nurse or other medical caregiver, such as the online service Blues On Call—or ask the company where you work if it has this service.

CHAPTER SIX

Imaging:
Asking the Right Questions

The dilemma

You get a chest X-ray because of a cough. The doctor tells you that the X-ray shows that your lungs are clear but that you have a spot on the bone of your left upper arm. He orders an MRI scan to check it out. After the MRI, the doctor says that further tests are necessary and wants to order a PET (positron emission tomography) scan. You are getting confused: Why so many tests?

A case study

Linda had a superficial skin cancer removed from her arm. She writes:

> *Well, yesterday I finally got the final results of all my tests. First of all, they don't usually do PET scans for squamous cell skin cancer, but since there is a study being done, I could have the scan at no cost to me. I was approved to be in it. We already knew that a PET scan shows up things that are not cancer, so when it showed something in my right calf, left elbow and neck, no one was terribly concerned. Because of the positive scan, I was scheduled to see the oncologist, who, being very cautious, ordered three MRIs of my leg and neck and an X-ray of the elbow. (All this extra*

expense! Poor Medicare.) Subsequently, all of these additional tests were interpreted as not showing any evidence of the spread of cancer.

The patient's point of view

Linda went to her nurse practitioner with an area of inflammation on her arm. Her NP told her it looked like cancer and surgically removed it. The pathology report confirmed that it was cancer. Linda was understandably tense when her nurse gave her the pathology report. Like anyone in this situation, she wanted answers: How serious was it? Had the cancer spread to other places? Though the chance of this kind of cancer spreading is very small, Linda agreed to a scan.

What started as the simple surgical removal of a superficial skin cancer became much more complicated, involving repeated trips for extra scans and doctor appointments. In the process Linda was exposed to radiation, and she was inconvenienced by the amount of time necessary for follow-up.

In the end, all the tests were negative. Was it all worth it? It's difficult to say. It's hard to put a price tag on peace of mind, and some of these tests provide that. In such circumstances, most patients will readily agree with their doctor's recommendation for further tests. If you find yourself in a similar situation, at the very least you should talk with your physician about the accuracy of the test and what can be learned from it.

'At the very least you should talk with your physician about the accuracy of the test and what can be learned from it.'

The doctor's point of view

When confronting the possibility of cancer or other serious illness, the doctor feels the patient's tension and the need to move expeditiously in getting a definite diagnosis. Cost is generally not discussed, though the tests are expensive.

In ordering diagnostic tests, both doctors and patients need to know the incidence of false positives and false negatives. A "false positive" is just what it sounds like: a positive test result when the disease or condition is *not* present. A false negative is a negative test result when the disease or condition *is* present. A positive test result will usually require more tests to determine if the test is a false positive or not. Occasionally one test leads to another test so that the technology seems to take on a life of its own. Decisions about diagnostic and treatment plans may be made on the basis of what technology is available.

Advances in technology

When I started medical practice in 1965, essentially everything I could do for a patient I could do out of my doctor's bag. We had no respiratory therapists, no physiotherapists, intensive care units, or the many other highly trained and specialized workers in diagnosis and treatment. Along with these changes came technological advances that saved lives and restored function. We now have machines that can peer into body cavities, permitting diagnoses that were mostly educated guesswork years ago. We have treatment modalities (dialysis machines and ventilators, for example) that extend life.

Most of us wouldn't want to go back in time, but we must be aware that diagnostic tests and scans are not infallible and can result in false positives and false negatives.

In the PET scan, radioactive glucose is injected into the bloodstream of the patient. Glucose or sugar is the essential substance burned by the body for energy. The PET scanner measures the radioactivity coming from all areas of the body. Areas where there is an accumulation of glucose will "light up" on the scan. The areas indicate points of increased metabolism of glucose. Cancer cells metabolize more rapidly, and cancerous areas will generally show on the scan. The careful doctor will then do further tests to verify the findings.

The problem is that PET scans are not specific for cancer. *Any* area that takes up more glucose will show up on a scan. Non-cancerous problems, such as inflammation and infection may look like cancer, resulting in a false positive. Since the spot on the scan cannot be distinguished from cancer, further tests often become necessary.

As in Linda's story above, a false-positive test will add considerably to the cost of care, in addition to the inconvenience and risk inherent in more tests.

Remember ...

When your doctor suggests that a scan be done, be prepared to ask questions and do some research on the Internet. Scans can be falsely positive or falsely negative as described above. Anytime diagnostic tests are ordered, the risk of the test must be weighed against the likelihood that it will yield useful information. Avoid the tendency to agree to a test or scan "because my insurance will cover it." There are specific times when it's a good idea to pause, take a deep breath and ask questions. It isn't necessarily in your best interest to do another procedure simply because it *can* be done.

What you can do to ask the right questions about tests

1. Following is a partial list of questions to ask when facing a diagnostic test:
    a) What specifically do we intend to learn from the test?
    b) How is the test done, and what (if any) are the risks of doing the test?
    c) How accurate is the test? What is the chance the test will be positive even though there is no disease or abnormal condition? What is the chance the test will be negative even though I have the condition?
    d) What do we do if the test is positive?
    e) What do we do if the test is negative?
    f) How much does the test cost?
    g) How much (if any) of the cost of the test is covered by my insurance?
2. Take time to evaluate the answers during an open discussion with your doctor.
3. Check out the AHRQ (Agency for Healthcare Research and Quality) that suggests you build a customized list of questions to ask in different situations. Visit *http://www.ahrq.gov/questionsaretheanswer/question.*

CHAPTER SEVEN

Second Opinion:
When Should You Get One?

The dilemma

You have an old hip injury, and over the last five years the pain has become constant. Your difficulty walking is affecting your work. At age 55, your primary care doctor tells you that you're too young for a joint replacement. You have a friend who had a hip replacement and is pain free and walks well. You would like the opinion of an orthopedic surgeon but your doctor hasn't suggested a consultation and you don't want to offend him by requesting a second opinion. It seems disrespectful to your doctor who has given you good care over the years. What can you do?

Sam—in his own words

I was 28 years old when I was diagnosed with cancer of the testicle at a nearby regional medical center. The cancer had already spread to my lungs. The testicle was removed and I was treated with chemotherapy. Subsequently the cancer reappeared in the incision of the former surgery. This was treated with intense radiation. As a result of the radiation my femoral artery closed and I had several operations to try to open or bypass the blocked-off artery. My leg was weak but the cancer was gone.

Seventeen years later, at age 45, I noticed a lump in the groin area that had been radiated. A biopsy showed this to be a sarcoma, a cancer caused by the previous radiation. I attended a conference with five doctors—including a surgeon, an orthopedist and a pathologist—to discuss further treatment. I was impressed that five doctors sat down in one room and spent time on my case. They said that with this kind of cancer they needed to take it out with a wide margin around the tumor. Their recommendation was a hemipelvectomy, which meant taking off my leg and half of my pelvis. A date for surgery was set in three weeks.

I went home and stomped around the kitchen and cried. I didn't want a quarter of my body lopped off. I felt that with this operation I could no longer function as a pastor. Then I remembered that an X-ray technician at the medical center had said I had a rare type of tumor, and that they only saw about four per year. After talking with a cardiologist doctor friend, I decided to get another opinion. My doctors at the medical center said, "That is your choice."

I was able to get an appointment at Memorial Sloan Kettering Cancer Center. With the doctors' permission, I collected all my lab, scan and pathology reports. The surgeon at Sloan Kettering said they saw four cases of sarcoma per week. After he examined my records, he informed me that the massive surgery was not necessary. He subsequently took out the tumor and, in the next six months, I had local radiation implants and chemotherapy.

In the 13 years since my surgery, all my tests showed no evidence of cancer. My leg is weak, but I can walk and continue my work. People say that I'm a miracle.

It was hard to decide to get a second opinion. I felt like I was slapping my doctors in the face. They had taken good care of me, and I didn't want to hurt their feelings or damage their professional pride. But when I heard that my tumor was rarely seen at the regional center, and when I considered how life-changing the operation would be, I decided I needed to get a second opinion. I thought, after all, I am the patient here.

The patient's point of view

Sam was understandably deeply distressed, feeling that the recommended disfiguring surgery would leave him disabled and possibly unable to continue his work as a pastor. Yet Sam, like many people, was reluctant to see another doctor for a second opinion. He felt loyalty to the doctors who had cared for him the previous 17 years with his first cancer. However, when Sam considered the extent of the operation and the fact that this medical center saw his type of tumor only rarely, he decided to get another opinion. It was appropriate for him to say, "*I* am the patient here" because he would be the one who would have to live with the results of the radical surgery and subsequent disability.

Other patients have other reasons for seeking a second opinion. Certain diseases may have a *confusing* set of symptoms. A consultation with another doctor or specialist may move the diagnosis process forward or may significantly change the course of treatment. In addition, any patient who is told that his or her situation is *hopeless* should consider another opinion. A second opinion also should be sought when a case is considered *borderline*—when it's unclear whether the treatment would help *or* if it's unclear whether the potential benefits of a treatment outweigh the attendant risks.

In cases with multiple and confusing symptoms, patients may find themselves referred from one specialist to another—and then yet another. In this situation, *the patient needs a healthcare advocate*, a medically knowledgeable person who can help to sort out the details of diagnosis and treatment. The most logical person for this role is the primary care physician, but a nurse or other healthcare professional also could help. In Sam's case, his cardiologist friend served as an advocate.

The doctor's point of view

It is said that in medical school the student learns the common presentation of common diseases. The remainder of a physician's career, it is said, is devoted to learning the uncommon presentation of common diseases and the common presentation of uncommon diseases. (Are you still with me?!)

The issue of a second opinion comes up in difficult cases with uncommon presentations or in cases of uncommon diseases. Confusing lab tests or other test results may obscure the way forward to a diagnosis. Or there may be questions about the relative risk of a surgery compared with the hoped-for benefit. Most doctors are open to the suggestion of a second opinion—or may *themselves* suggest a second opinion. Your physician will generally know where to go for a specific problem and can help you find the proper consultant. Keep in mind, though, as in Sam's case, it's advisable to do some investigation on your own.

'Most doctors are open to the suggestion of a second opinion—or may *themselves* suggest a second opinion.'

Primary care physicians who refer patients to a specialist want to hear about the outcome of the second consultation. After getting a second opinion, remind the consulting doctor to make sure the referring doctor gets a copy of the findings and recommendations.

Remember ...

By openly discussing your desire for a second opinion, your doctor can cooperate fully in forwarding records that will aid the consultant or specialist. If your doctor is reluctant to cooperate in finding a consultant, check with centers that deal with the kind of problem you have. Large regional clinics are accustomed to receiving patients with confusing or perplexing medical problems and can facilitate a consultation with an appropriate staff member. Remember that you are entitled to copies of your medical records, and it is essential that your consulting doctor makes these records available. The right to access to one's medical records is mandated by provisions of the Health Insurance Portability and Accountability Act (HIPAA) enacted by Congress in 1996.

What you can do when a second opinion may be called for

1. Be aware that in specific medical situations a second opinion should be sought:
    *   When you are told the case is hopeless

- When there is difficulty or delay in establishing a diagnosis
- When there is question of whether the potential benefits of a procedure outweigh the risks
- When a condition is not improving
- When you are diagnosed with a rare condition that requires the services of a specialist in that field
- When your research about your chronic disease suggests you may not be getting the most appropriate treatment
- When an opinion from a doctor in a different specialty is needed (for example, consultation with an oncologist after cancer surgery)
- When there's a question about the need for a procedure for a patient with a terminal disease
- When a patient is in a terminal condition and the doctor suggests that he or she should be moved to intensive care

2. Cultivate open communication with your primary care physician so that the possibility of a second opinion can be discussed openly.
3. Prepare for the second-opinion consultation by assembling all pertinent records, including lab, X-ray, scan, and pathology reports, along with the reports of previous procedures, as well as clinical notes.
4. Make certain your primary care physician receives a report of the consultation.

CHAPTER EIGHT

Pre-Planning:
Who Will Speak for You?

The dilemma

Your 87-year-old mother is getting forgetful; sometimes you question her mental capabilities. When your father died eight years ago after a stroke, your family went through tense times as you made the decision to have a feeding tube inserted, a situation that continued for a number of months. You wonder what it will be like if you and your brother and sister have to make similar decisions for your mother. What can you do?

Case study: Why are they doing this?

Joe was an interesting character with colorful language who started smoking as a teenager. After five decades, the smoking caught up with him, and Joe began having trouble breathing. When he could no longer walk up the short hill to his house, Joe sought medical attention and was found to have emphysema. Joe tried to quit smoking but never quite stopped. Gradually his breathing problem became worse and finally he needed oxygen at home.

One day I got a call from Joe's wife who said she had called the EMT (emergency medical technician) squad because Joe couldn't breathe. She said the

EMTs had placed a tube in Joe's windpipe and were on their way to the ER. I told her I would meet them there.

When I arrived at the hospital, Joe's wife was angry. She said, "Why are they doing this to Joe? He has been suffering terribly for the past months, and it would be better if we just let him go." As gently as I could, I told her that when the paramedics are called they can't make those judgments. They do what they're trained to do; they get the emergency situation under control and take the patient to the hospital. Prior to this episode, Joe and his wife had never discussed end-of-life issues.

In the hospital Joe's breathing improved. He was discharged after eight days and sent home with a visiting nurse. He died at home three weeks later.

Because of Joe's experience, I made it a point to discuss end-of-life issues with my elderly patients and with those who had incurable diseases. Thereafter, I kept a list of names in my office of people who specifically said they did not want to be resuscitated in case of a cardiac arrest. In each case, I asked that they talk to their spouse, their children and their pastor about their wishes.

Case study: unexpected decisions

A 66-year-old man, "Herb," was admitted to the hospital with cancer of the pancreas, which had been diagnosed three months earlier. Since that time Herb was in almost constant pain and lost considerable weight. He was unable to eat or take liquids for the last two days.

After Herb was admitted, lab tests showed that his kidneys were no longer functioning properly. The hospital doctors (I wasn't directly involved in this case) advised moving Herb to the intensive care unit where they planned to start kidney dialysis. The doctors came to the family members for their approval before moving Herb to the ICU.

Herb had not formulated "advance directives" that stated his preferences or any limitations with regard to his healthcare.

The family's point of view

When a spouse or adult children are suddenly faced with making a decision that affects the immediate future of their loved one, how that decision is made and who makes it will depend on how the family has functioned in the past. Ordinarily, if the spouse is living and capable, he or she will be the primary person making the decision. If there is tension among family members, making these decisions can be very disruptive to relationships. Even when an elderly loved one has a terminal illness, many families avoid the difficult discussions until the situation becomes critical.

The lack of communication among family members can complicate the medical care of the loved one and add unnecessary discomfort and cost.

I had an elderly patient "Edith," who lived in a nursing home and had been confused for many years. One of Edith's daughters was very attentive and visited faithfully every week. When Edith got sick with a lung infection, she was hospitalized with pneumonia.

In consultation with her daughter, we treated Edith with antibiotics but with defined limitations. Several days later another daughter, who hadn't seen her mother in five years, arrived from out of state and emphatically insisted on intensive treatment. As a result, Edith lived another 10 days before she died. The cost to Medicare for those 10 days was well in excess of $10,000.

The doctor's point of view

In Herb's story above, the doctors knew that unless more intensive efforts were made, Herb would die soon. The physicians let the family know that Herb needed dialysis to prolong his life. In end-of-life situations, most doctors won't be specific in trying to predict the outcome of an intervention or how long a life will be prolonged. They also will want to be careful not to promise that, by prolonging life, an underlying problem, such as Herb's cancer, will improve.

A doctor may have ideas and even convictions about what should be done in a terminal case, but the decision for or against more intensive treatment must be that of the patient and/or individuals representing the patient. Doctors will present possible measures to prolong life, even though they may believe that these measures are not advisable and that they will only prolong the misery of a dying patient. When I, as a physician, was faced with this situation, I felt the need to remain neutral. Patients and their families understood this but would sometimes ask what I would do if it were a member of my family. I would then try to answer truthfully.

Advance directives

In the event that you aren't able to speak for yourself, advance directives are a written record of your instructions to the people who are making healthcare decisions on your behalf. Advance directives have two parts: (1) A "living will" gives instructions on your wishes regarding limitations on using life-sustaining measures, such as CPR (cardiopulmonary resuscitation), assisted breathing, and feeding tubes. (2) The "power of attorney for healthcare decisions" appoints a spokesperson for a group of people, such as the patient's adult children, who will make healthcare decisions when a patient is incapacitated.

State laws vary somewhat with regard to advance directives. All states, however, have accepted the concept that the wishes of the individual who has formulated advance directives need to be respected. (See Chapter 21 for more information on advance directives.) The American Hospital Association, along with other organizations, has an excellent discussion of the need for, and practical suggestions about, drawing up advance directives. Access the site at *http://www.putitinwriting.org/putitinwriting_app/content/ piiwbrochure.pdf.*

'The end of a parent's life
can be made more tragic by
bad decision making, *or* it can
unite a family in new ways.'

Remember ...

The need for families to make healthcare decisions for their parents is a common occurrence. It's a time of tension and uncertainty. If adult children and their parents discuss these issues *before* a healthcare crisis occurs, parents will be more at ease. If adult children hear and agree to respect their parents' wishes, the way through difficult decision making will become smoother and less tense—though such issues, of course, are never easy. The end of a parent's life can be made more tragic by bad decision making, *or* it can unite a family in new ways. For an example of a positive end-of-life story, see Chapter 17 about my father's care—and his decisions—at the end of his life.

What you can do to plan for your passing

1. Consider possible limits to your treatment. Specifically put it in writing if you do not want:
   - CPR if you experience cardiac arrest
   - To be placed on a ventilator (with a machine that keeps you breathing)
   - A feeding tube in the event you cannot eat or swallow
   - Other life-sustaining measures when it has been determined that you have terminal cancer or irreversible, severe brain damage
2. Check out the specific requirements of your state for advance directives at: *http://www.uslivingwillregistry. com/forms.shtm* or *http://www.noah-health.org/en/rights/endoflife/ adforms.html*.
3. Discuss your wishes with your family and any others who will make decisions in the event you're unable to do so.
4. Send a copy of your advance directives to your doctor, family members, spiritual/religious adviser and attorney.

5. Be prepared to ask the questions appropriate to the situation. For example, these are the kinds of questions the family might be asking in Herb's story above:
    - What is his approximate life expectancy with regard to the cancer?
    - Is the transfer to ICU necessary to prolong his life?
    - What will be done in the ICU that is not now being done?
    - Can he be expected to regain the same status or condition as before the pneumonia?
    - Will we be able to see him in the ICU?
    - Will he be more comfortable there than in a regular hospital room?
    - Can we place limits on the extent of his care? For example, can we agree to and sign a DNR (do not resuscitate) order?
    - If we agree to place him on assisted ventilation, how do we decide when to take him off?
    - Should (can) we consult another doctor for another opinion?
    - Might it be best to transfer him to hospice care? And if so, when and under what circumstances?

CHAPTER NINE

Wellness:
You *Become* Your Choices

The dilemma

Most of us, if we sit in a quiet place and honestly ask our-selves, "What can I do to feel better, to be healthier and to improve my chances of living longer?" can immediately come up with at least three or four things. It's not that we don't know what we can do to be healthier; it's just that we don't get around to *doing* it. How can we change?

Case study 1: George

In May 2005 "George" was more than 70 pounds overweight. His blood lipids (cholesterol, triglyc-erides, etc.) were high, his blood pressure was ele-vated and he had diabetes. He was taking four medicines for these conditions, plus stool softener and thyroid medicine. At today's prices his drug bill would be more than $2,400 a year.

George entered a weight-reduction program and, one year later, he was near his ideal weight. During that year, as he lost weight, George also dropped his med-icines one by one. By May 2006, George no longer needed any medication. In addition, George didn't need to spend money checking his sugars at home, and he no longer needed the quarterly office visits to monitor his diabetes, blood pressure and kidney func-tion. Today George remains disease-free.

The patient's point of view

George suffered from a group of symptoms so common that it has a name: metabolic syndrome. People with the metabolic syndrome are at increased risk of coronary heart disease, stroke, peripheral artery disease and Type 2 diabetes. Metabolic syndrome has become increasingly common in the United States, afflicting more than 50 million people (nearly one-sixth of the total U.S. population).

With proper diet and weight reduction, George's diabetes and high blood pressure disappeared. He saved money on his medications, blood tests and medical office visits. More importantly, people like George who make these kinds of adjustments have more energy and a better sense of self. George can reasonably expect to live longer and with more vigor as a result of his choices and actions.

For many of us, it's not that we don't know what to do, we just don't *do*. We know we eat too much, eat the wrong things, exercise too little, get less sleep than recommended, smoke or drink too much, overuse prescription meds, and/or don't set aside time to renew our minds and spirits. In short, we procrastinate. (See Chapter 25 for more on procrastination. You *do* plan to read Chapter 25, don't you? Without delay?!)

Case studies 2 and 3: Melanie and Elizabeth

Melanie came to see me with complaints of nervousness and inability to sleep. She appeared tense and twitchy. I asked her about her eating and sleeping habits. She said she drank three pots of coffee per day, smoked two packs of cigarettes each day and slept about four hours a night. This information was elicited only through specific questions. It apparently had never occurred to Melanie that these habits alone could account for her symptoms.

Elizabeth came to the office for a routine follow-up visit. I asked her what she does for exercise. She said that every day she moves her limbs and back through a full range of motion. She offered to show me her exercise routine and proceeded to demonstrate on the floor of the exam room. I was impressed that she indeed moved all her joints through a full range of motion. Elizabeth was 92 years old. When I complimented her she said very simply, "It always made sense to me that if I wanted my joints to continue to move properly, all I needed to do was to keep them moving." I am convinced she was right.

The doctor's point of view

Traditionally, the doctor's role has been about treating disease and not about promoting health. When a patient comes to a doctor with a complaint—such as pain, fever or weakness—the doctor's task has been to get that patient back to where he or she no longer suffers from the symptoms.

In my own practice, I found that promoting good healthy lifestyles tended to be frustrating with most patients. When they appeared at the office for a complete physical, I usually had their lab tests in hand. After taking a detailed history and doing a physical exam, I went over the findings, including the lab tests. The remainder of the time was spent in giving them ideas and information about how they could improve their current health, as well as their prospects for good health in the future. More often than not, when patients returned six months or a year later, they had followed only some—or even none—of my recommendations.

How was I to interpret this? These experiences verified for me how difficult it is for most of us to take the long view and make changes that will improve our chances for a healthy and happy old age. Rather, we want reassurance that there is no immediate threat to our health and current lifestyle.

Doctors also are constrained by the fact that they aren't compensated financially for the time they spend in wellness and preventive healthcare. Doing a blood-pressure check takes less time than counseling a patient on lifestyle changes. With the emphasis on curative—not preventive—medicine, there's generally little financial return for spending extra time with a patient on wellness issues.

Wellness is a choice

Wellness starts with a can-do attitude that sheds the idea that I am a victim of my circumstances. Rather, I acknowledge that many things *are* under my control: *I* am the one who decides, for starters, what goes into my mouth. In order to control the things that affect my health, I need to be educated on the issues where I can positively influence my health and longevity. Then, with that understanding, I can take responsibility to make the necessary changes. The rewards are more energy, a more positive outlook, and an improved chance of living a long and productive life.

'Wellness starts with a can-do attitude that sheds the idea that I am a victim of my circumstances.'

Remember …

A few decades ago a book was published under the title *You Are What You Eat*. Well, in like manner you *become* the choices you make. If you choose to overeat, you will in all likelihood become overweight, less physically active, and more prone to diabetes, high blood pressure, heart attacks, and a reduced life span. You have control over many things—including food intake—that will affect your self-image, self-esteem and outlook on life. The rewards go to those who make good lifestyle choices for the long haul, people like Elizabeth in the story above.

What you can do to enhance your health and wellness

1. Sit under a tree or on your favorite chair with no TV, no radio and no interruptions and, either individually or with family or a trusted friend, reflect on the specific steps you can take to live a healthier life. Remember that health includes not only the physical, but also the mental, emotional and spiritual. Write down these steps and action plans.
    a) Start with only two or three items, no more. What information do you need to get started?
    b) How do you arrange your time so as to provide the space to attend to the issues you identified?
    c) How will you know that you are succeeding? Try to identify specific evaluation or monitoring techniques.
    d) Where will you find encouragement and accountability to persist? (With whom can you do this activity?)
    e) How will you reward yourself—and celebrate—when you achieve a goal?

2. Make sure that your first goals are both realistic and doable. Later you can identify and work at more advanced goals and objectives.

3. Read about procrastination and learn to recognize when you are procrastinating.

4. Get educated on what is within your power to change that will in turn improve your health, such as:

    • Weight loss to achieve your optimal weight (body mass index less than 25 kg/m2); see BMI calculator at *http://www.jennycraig.com/etools/yourstyle/?dfa=1.*

    • Increased physical activity, with a goal of at least 30 minutes of moderately intense activity at least three days a week.

    • Healthful eating habits that include reduced intake of saturated fats, trans fats and cholesterol. If and when you overeat, reflect on why. Is food a substitute for something missing or unresolved in your life? You might want to consider counseling if that would help you gain a deeper understanding of what makes you tick.

5. Believe that the positive changes you make are not just for a few weeks or months but for the rest of your life with counseling if that would help you gain a deeper understanding of what makes you tick.

CHAPTER TEN

Complementary and Alternative Medicine: Is There Another Way?

The dilemma

What do you do when your child is sick and not improving with treatment from the best available doctors? You have heard good reports of the benefits of seeing a naturopath, but you wonder about taking your child to a practitioner of alternative medicine. What should you do?

Case study

In his first year of life, "Matthew" had recurrent episodes of bronchiolitis and pneumonia that required frequent visits to the pediatrician and occasionally to the emergency room. He was treated with antibiotics, bronchodilators and several short-term doses of steroids.

At age 3, after starting pre-school, Matthew again got a severe cold that developed into a cough and lung congestion. The cold lasted two months despite treatment with antibiotics and nebulized bronchodilators. When Matthew's symptoms persisted, his pediatrician added nebulized steroids. On the advice of the pediatrician, Matthew's mother ("Jan") consulted an allergist who continued the treatment as before. When

Matthew still didn't improve, Jan took him two weeks later to a lung specialist who also made no changes in treatment.

Jan noticed a marked personality change in her young son. He became aggressive and irritable. His hair was falling out, and he complained of pain in his head and stomach. Jan checked on the side effects of the medicines and became convinced that these changes were related to the steroids he was taking. Jan stopped the steroids and, within two days, her son again became "the same sweet boy I knew." Jan knew there must be another option in how to treat the lung problem.

Jan took Matthew to see a doctor of naturopathy who spent 90 minutes taking a detailed history of the course of the boy's illness, including diet, activities and living environment. Matthew's family history was not available since he was adopted. The doctor pre-scribed changes in his diet, increased vitamin C and anti-oxidants, and ordered a tincture to clear his lungs. Matthew's lung problem improved in two days.

The naturopathic doctor called several times to check on Matthew's condition but saw him only once. The total cost of her services was about $200. Six weeks later Jan took her son to his pediatrician who was delighted to find Matthew's lungs were clear. Years later Matthew has had no recurrence of these prob-lems. Jan continues to take Matthew to see his pedia-trician for care and advice.

The patient's point of view

Young Matthew had a persistent problem with his lungs. After seeing no improvement from the conventionally prescribed medicines—and with evidence of disturbing side effects—Jan took Matthew to a doctor of naturopathy. Naturopathy is one of the disciplines considered part of complementary and alternative medicine (CAM).[7]

There are many reasons why people turn to CAM. The cost of conventional medicine is high and escalating much faster than wages and the inflation rate. People look for less expensive alternatives. When an illness lingers on, helpful friends tell stories of how they benefited from various sources, including CAM practitioners. Other patients who have been told they have an incurable illness seek CAM practitioners as a source of hope in an otherwise hopeless situation. Jan appreciated the amount of time and careful listening by the naturopath at the time of Matthew's visit.

> *Some patients choose to integrate CAM with conventional therapy. Jean was such a person. A nurse-turned-artist, she was diagnosed at age 55 with multiple myeloma. Her doctors told her that the disease was in its early stages and that any chemotherapy was premature. Jean and her husband were not comfortable to sit idly by as the disease progressed. They learned from alternative newsletters of treatment designed to invoke the immune system to resist the progression. Over a period of years she went for testing and received injections. Her oncologists were fully informed of the alternative therapy she was receiving, and Jean cooperated fully with her physicians in subsequent chemotherapy. The alternative therapy was in addition to the standard treatment.*

The doctor's point of view

Traditional or conventional doctors believe that their care of patients is scientifically proven to be effective. Any treatment or drug must go through a series of pre-clinical testing and eventual testing on a large group of patients using a "double blind" method to rule out the placebo effect, as well as to assess effectiveness and incidence of undesirable side effects. A placebo is a substance that has no pharmacological effect—a "sugar pill"—but produces a desired result through psychological or other unknown mechanisms. A placebo may approach the same rate of effectiveness as the active ingredient, depending on the condition being tested and the design of the test.

So doctors are skeptical of methods of treatment that haven't gone through the same kind of evaluation. They know that in the absence of scientific evidence of the effectiveness of a drug or treatment, practitioners take a risk of censure from their professional organization or a lawsuit from their patient for using unproven methods.

Doctors also need to recognize, however, that conventional medicine is far from infallible. Drug reactions with untoward side effects are always a possibility when there's an unusual response to a drug. One of my roles as a consulting internist was to take patients *off* their medicines.

Doctors also know that conventional medicine doesn't have answers to all healthcare problems. It presents a dilemma when a patient for whom the doctor has nothing further to suggest for treatment comes asking the doctor's opinion about seeing a CAM practitioner (see Chapter 22 for further discussion of this issue).

Can a CAM treatment come into the mainstream?

There is a catch-22 dilemma in the issue of CAM research. CAM is said to lack the scientific evidence that it works, but the accuser (that is, the conventional healthcare system) controls the money given out in grants that would allow the research to prove or disprove the effectiveness of a particular CAM. Until recently, money for research grants for CAM studies was controlled by the proponents of traditional medicine and not available to CAM practitioners. Increasingly, though, medical schools in the United States are developing departments of complementary and alternative medicine, finally making some funds available for adequate research. Recognizing that full acceptance will come only with objective, scientific evidence, researchers with an interest in CAM continue to devise the necessary studies to prove its efficacy.

As specific CAM methods are found to be effective, they are transferred from the list of unproven methods to approved treatments. It should be noted that many of our present medicines started out as unproven alternative medicines that were later proven to be effective.

'Many of our present medicines started out as unproven alternative medicines that were later proven to be effective.'

Remember ...

Complementary and alternative medicine methods frequently lack scientific proof of their effectiveness. Hearsay evidence and advertisements may be misleading. The hoped-for benefits from any CAM treatment must be weighed against the potential to do harm. When considering CAM, the Internet and other sources of information should be consulted. Remember to inform your primary care physician about any CAM treatment you are trying.

What you can do with regard to complementary and alternative medicine

1. When you or your child are being treated by conventional medicine for a condition and continue to have troubling symptoms, consider the possibility that the symptoms may be a reaction to the medicine.
2. Check the Internet and other sources for evidence of the effectiveness of a CAM treatment, but don't depend on advertisements or websites for your information. Check these websites for more information on CAM and how to evaluate a website that advertises health remedies: *http://nccam.nih.gov* and *http://nccam.nih.gov/health/webresources/*.
3. Be alert to the possibility that the CAM practitioner (or conventional practitioner, for that matter) is fraudulent and a "quack" (see the defining traits of a quack in Chapter 22).
4. Discuss with your primary care physician the possibility of seeing a CAM practitioner. Your doctor can tell you if your condition is likely to be helped with a CAM treatment and also can discuss with you the potential for harm from the CAM treatment. It should be noted that some conventional doctors are more open to CAM and some are less open. If your doctor is not open and if integration

of the two is important to you (like Jean above), you may need to change doctors.

5. Notify your doctor of any CAM treatment you are taking in addition to conventional treatment.

PART II

Reshaping the Doctor Image— Personal Stories

CHAPTER ELEVEN

The Fading Doctor Mystique

More than 60 years ago while playing basketball I jumped for a rebound and came down on someone else's foot. There was a loud crack and immediate pain. My mother thought I may have broken a bone and called Doctor Devonthal. He had been our family physician for many years at times of childbirth, appendicitis and my brother's "spasms" caused by a milk allergy. Dr. Devonthal's word was law when an illness struck; his instructions were unquestioningly followed.

So when Dr. Devonthal said my ankle problem was just a sprain, this diagnosis was accepted without question—and even without an X-ray. We followed his directions, and the ankle healed.

When I was a lad, doctors like Dr. Devonthal were thought to be special, set-apart people. The doctor was one of the few educated people in my community. As a consequence, he was often sought after for more than his medical expertise (and, yes, doctors in those days were almost always male). He was essential to running the local hospital, he served as chairman of the school board and the library board, and he was counselor to local politicians and bankers.

At the mid-point of the 20th century there was a mystique—even a sense of mystery—that surrounded doctors. They knew things about the human body that were incomprehensible and unknowable to just about everyone else. Most people viewed them with awe and wonder. Their power to heal was shrouded in mystery. With much of what went wrong with the human body beyond knowing, a blind faith in the ability of the doctor to bring about healing was a basic requirement in the doctor-patient relationship. The doctor was the adult, the patient was the child—and all that was needed from the patients was that they be able to follow directions for the prescribed treatment. There was no questioning of the diagnosis and no discussion of alternative treatments.

'It was as if she had met a head of state that night.'

To some people, physicians were not an ordinary part of the human race. After I became a doctor, I was interested in this phenomenon. My patient Earl, a gentleman in his 70s, apparently could not see me as anything other than his doctor. At church I was careful not to ask Earl the customary, "How are you?" because 20 minutes later I would have received a detailed accounting of how all of his bodily systems were functioning. At least that's the way it seemed to me. One late evening on my way home from a medical meeting, I stopped at a filling station for gasoline. A young woman at the next pump kept glancing my way with particular intensity. As I completed my task, she turned to me and gushed, "You're Dr. Miller, aren't you?" It was as if she had met a head of state that night. On another occasion a woman standing behind me in a hospital cafeteria line said in apparent wonder at a new and astounding truth, "Doctors eat *too*?" (She wasn't joking.) I mumbled a reply, although I was tempted to say, "Yes, and I also go to the bathroom."

The patient as knowledgeable partner

As I write this, all of that seems quaint and from a bygone era. So much has changed. For one thing, the education of doctors has changed—and that education assumes the patient is much more knowledgeable than in the past. This has been a gradual process for most people. Increasingly, doctors see their patients as having checked out the possibilities for diagnosis and treatment. The doctor is no longer the caring parent, and the patient is no longer the unknowing child. This is a drastically different relationship. What has changed is primarily the patient who now is a knowledgeable partner in his or her healthcare instead of the blindly trusting child figure.

In the last 10 to 15 years, medical information has become easily accessible with the advent and wide availability of the Internet. Merck Manual at *http://www.merck.com/mmpe/index.html* and WebMD at *http://www.webmd.com/* are excellent examples of this. At the WebMD site, you are led through a program that, after you describe your symptoms, lists possible diagnoses. For example, if you say you have sharp, lower-right abdominal pain, a list of 20 diagnoses appears, led by appendicitis, with an explanation of its causes, its symptoms and its treatment. *Merck Manual* gives similar detailed descriptions of many diseases and conditions.

This new relationship can best be described as collaborative, one with open and free communication. Upon entering into this collaboration, the doctor has rejoined the human race, just one more mortal—albeit with specialized information that can benefit the patient.

'This new relationship can best be described as collaborative, one with open and free communication.'

Encounters between doctor and patient were discussed in detail with a focus group of consumers of healthcare. One person, and to varying degrees several others in the group, could not *imagine* engaging her doctor in the kind of communication necessary to achieve the goals of this book. At the end of the eight-week period, all members of the group specifically said they felt comfortable talking to at least *this* doctor, the author of *Empowering the Patient.* That's a start.

It's time for the doctor mystique to fade from view, much as the telegraph and the typewriter have outlived their usefulness. The following chapters center on themes from my own experience. It is my hope that this personal telling will help individuals see their doctor and other healthcare provider as *persons*—not as categories or caricatures—real people who are available to them to maximize their lives and help them reach their God-given potential for health and wholeness.

CHAPTER TWELVE

Motivated to Serve

I grew up in a family of nine children during the Great Depression. As a pre-teen in rural Ohio, I recall seeing the occasional hobo walking along the road with halting gait and ragged clothes. Usually my mother sent a couple of us children out to him with a plate of food. He was an object of curiosity, nothing more.

For our family to survive the hard times, we had to stick together. It was assumed that the needs of the family came before any individual needs. Deferring to one another was necessary and a way of life. Beginning at age 13, each summer I worked for my uncle, helping make hay or other farm work. My uncle wanted no idle hands. One time during a break from making hay, he told me, "While you're resting, move that pile of bricks to the back of the barn." At the end of each week, I turned over the money I earned to my father. I was allowed to keep one-eighth of the money; the rest went to sustain the family. I never questioned the system. It was the way things were done.

At the age of 12, I read a book that changed my life. I have no idea where the book *Dr. York, Hill Doctor* came from or how it came into my possession. I read the entire book practically in one sitting. The next day I picked up the book again and read it a second time. Young Dr. York had left the comforts and well-heeled confines of a large city to go to the hills of eastern Kentucky to provide medical care to people who had none. After reading that book, I quietly decided I wanted to be like Dr. York. (I have looked for that book since, without success.)

At first I told no one of my aspirations to become a doctor, not even my parents. I knew that my cousins would have looked at me with derision for harboring such a ridiculous notion. Later, at a family gathering, my mother was asked which one of her boys was going to be a doctor. She pointed to me and said, "He *thinks* he is." I understood. It was presumptuous for a farm boy, raised during the Great Depression, to think of (much less verbalize) such a lofty goal. In that era doctors were revered with a level of respect that made them near mythical beings.

> 'In that era doctors were revered
> with a level of respect
> that made them
> near mythical beings.'

Once, as my father was giving me a haircut in the basement of our home, I did speak to him about going to college. Dad said he didn't object to my going but that he couldn't help me financially. I never mentioned it again. After graduation from high school, I worked as an apprentice plumber for two years. I was then drafted during the Korean War and, following my Mennonite pacifist upbringing, I registered as a conscientious objector.

The journey begins

As an alternative to military service, I worked in a mental hospital as a ward orderly. My supervisors, at my request, assigned me to night duty. This allowed me to start my pre-medical coursework at Kent State University in northeastern Ohio. Coming from a small rural high school with 24 in my graduating class, I had little idea of my capabilities. But I decided to plunge in and was elated with all A's after the first quarter of study. By taking summer courses, I completed the pre-med studies in three years. It was a glorious day when I was accepted at Western Reserve School of Medicine, also in Ohio, in 1957.

Medical school was as rigorous as expected. Marilyn Oswald and I had married before medical school and, during those four years, had three children. There were added pressures because we never seemed to have enough money (I use "we" in this context because it is difficult to use the singular after 53 years of married life). Between babies, Marilyn worked as a part-time nurse. The last two years I "externed" as a med-ical student in a Good Samaritan Hospital that provided room and board and $50 per month. Thus we were able to control our debt level.

Following graduation and one year of internship, we volun-teered to go for two years to Haiti to work in a small hospital. Part of my motivation for going to Haiti was because I was keenly aware of those of my generation who had gone to Korea and fought. Some had died there. Serving in Haiti was an attempt to do my part in a small way. In retrospect, this seems to be the first installment on living out my goal as a 12-year-old to go into medicine to serve poor people.

'I found that service was pleasure'

The two years in Haiti put us in touch with some of the poor-est people in the world. We saw individuals struggle with the things we take for granted like food, clothes and a roof over our heads. And most Haitians did this with grace. We also got a picture of our own country from the viewpoint of Haitians, with its wealth and emphasis on consumerism and material- ism. We became determined to be known for who we are, not what we own.

After a year of postgraduate training in Family Practice, it was time to find a place to settle in and raise our four chil- dren. Our country home near Bellefontaine, Ohio, was an ideal setting for these purposes.

Ten years after we were married, I was ready to start medical practice. Up to that point we had lived in 13 places in 10 years. Moving had become a way of life. After six months, our small children wondered when we were going to move again. Our combined income for the first ten years of our marriage was slightly over $2,000 per year.

I soon discovered that being a doctor is also being in busi- ness. In private practice, there are costs. The electricity, office assistants, insurance and the building itself all needed to be paid. The only way to cover those costs was the income gen- erated from seeing patients. However, I recalled that one of my mentors had said, "Just be concerned about the quality of care you provide; the finances will follow."

How was I to know how much to charge for my services? I started practice with an older colleague with prices set at the low end of the community average. On the one hand, I did not need or want to get rich quickly, but neither did I want patients to come to me because I was cheaper. I tried to be sensitive to those who couldn't pay and several times sent let- ters to people who owed large bills stating that I was ready to reduce or even cancel their charges if they contacted me and explained their circumstances. Despite more than a hundred such letters, only one person ever came to discuss his bill.

'We decided it was time to separate our wants from our needs.'

I finished paying off my medical school debts about six years after graduation. Having spent two years in Haiti among the poorest people in the world, Marilyn and I wanted to remain sensitive to the needs of the poor. But in spite of gradually increasing income, at the end of each year, it seemed as if we really could have used about $2,000 more. We decided it was time to separate our wants from our needs. It became clear that if we allowed our material wants to guide us, there would never be enough. On the other hand, our needs were definable and limited.

Now in my eighth decade and looking back, there appears to be a pattern of one decision leading to another. I ask myself, *What is the common thread that runs through a life that became involved in widely varied activities, traveling to more than 40 countries and living overseas for more than eleven years in five countries?* What I do know is that my childhood formation growing up in a big family under my mother's gentle and compassionate tutelage, my father's core principles of honesty and integrity, and my identity within a strong Mennonite community have all contributed immeasurably.

Along the way, I found purpose, even joy, in the feeling that I was contributing to a better life for those with whom I came in contact. The words of Nobel Prize-winning Indian poet Rabindranath Tagore capture my feelings:

I slept and dreamed that life was pleasure,
I woke and saw that life was service,
I served and found that service was pleasure.

CHAPTER THIRTEEN

Room for Compassion
in the Doctor's Office

In medical school, we started Anatomy class in the middle of the first year. The rather aloof Anatomy professor talked to us as neophyte students about our feelings as we were preparing to go to Anatomy Lab for dissection of a human body. He said we needed to approach this scientifically with an objective approach that would take away the subliminal feeling of horror that came with cutting into a human body—and the idea that this could be *me* on the dissection table. This was my first installment among many in the process of removing emotions from the task of making decisions based on facts and science, not subjective feelings.

So, early in my medical career I wanted to project an image of calmness and professional competence that would give patients a reason to trust my medical judgments. This approach largely blocked any real emotional connection between me and my patients. Gradually, however, I learned (over a period of years) that I could be more open about *my* feelings without the patients losing confidence in me. I began to enjoy my contacts with patients more.

Several incidents helped me shift toward being more compassionate—and not being afraid to show it. Many years ago in my practice in Ohio a man came to see me with chest pain that suggested angina. A cardiogram indicated an impending heart attack. I talked to him about the problem, and he said he would do everything possible to deal with it because he was very much looking forward to watching his twin sons play on the high school basketball team. He was admitted to the hospital, but at that time there was little we could do in such a situation except try to minimize the devastating effects of the expected heart attack.

When I arrived at the hospital the next morning the man was having severe pain and subsequently went into cardiac arrest. We tried to resuscitate him with the still new technique of closed chest massage—to no avail. (There are now more effective ways to intervene and prevent heart attacks.) I dreaded the task of telling the family the sad news.

'I don't recall the exact words I used, but I do remember that I cried with them.'

As I went to the waiting area to talk to his wife and sons, I wondered how to tell them that their husband and father had just died. I don't recall the exact words I used, but I do remember that I cried with them. It somehow seemed to me at that time that allowing myself to show emotion helped the woman and her sons be a little better able to cope with the tragic news. And contrary to feeling that I had in some way compromised my professionalism, I felt I had more effectively related to the family.

Entering into family tragedy in Egypt

In 1979 I went to a hospital in Egypt to teach medical students and residents internal medicine. The hospital had sent out notices of my arrival, including a news item in the *Al-Ahram,* the major Cairo newspaper. My days were filled with teaching rounds in the mornings and consultations in the afternoons. People came from miles away to see the American doctor.

One afternoon a man arrived with his 15-year-old son. They had traveled a long distance from his remote village to the south. His son had been ill for a number of months and had already seen doctors in other clinics. So when the father heard about the American doctor coming (probably by reading the account in the Cairo newspaper), he gathered his resources and traveled for several days in hopes that I could help his son.

Much was riding on the outcome of the visit. The son, the family's oldest child, was the one who had recently been sent to school to get an education in the expectation that he would find good employment and thereby lift the family out of poverty. All members of the family had sacrificed their personal wants in order to pay for the education of the young man.

I asked the father the usual questions about how long his son had been sick, how the problem started and the nature of his symptoms. The boy looked as if he had been sick a long time. His skin and eyes were the jaundiced color of liver failure. His abdomen protruded like that of a term pregnancy. I began to examine him with a heavy heart because it was already clear to me that there was nothing anyone could do for him.

The youth had advanced liver cirrhosis and failure caused by schistosomiasis. The schistosome is a parasite whose intermediary host is the snails found in the canals of Egypt. The parasite enters the body of swimmers and eventually causes cirrhosis. His swollen abdomen was due to the scarred liver and the buildup of pressure of blood returning through the liver. Thirty years ago nothing could be done to cure this terminal illness.

While I was examining the boy, I became keenly aware of the father standing nearby, expectantly and eagerly awaiting the words that would assure him of his son's recovery. I struggled to find the words I knew I needed to say. As gently as I could through a translator, I gave the man the bad news. The earlier look of hope on the father's face literally dissolved into paroxysms of grief. For years thereafter I could not retell that story without weeping.

Thus on the one hand, I had been taught in my medical training to be objective and emotionally detached in order to make dispassionate decisions. On the other hand, I did not want to abandon the human race—or my own humanity—and lose all feeling and empathy.

> '"Patients will assume that
> you *know*; what they really
> want to know is if you *care*."'

In my medical practice, I gradually moved from the always serious professional to where I could engage in lighthearted humor and repartee, usually with colleagues but sometimes with patients and their families as well. Even in the face of devastating news, there was often room for optimism and hope, and I tried to communicate those qualities. In my own practice I attempted to follow the advice that I gave to young physicians: "Patients will assume that you *know*; what they really want to know is if you *care*."

Seeking the 'compassion balance' in India

Later, in India, I again faced the issue of empathy and my ability to function. Living in Calcutta in the early 1990s, the evidence of poverty—people living on the street, children without healthcare, families not knowing if they would have a next meal—all began to press in on me. We had previously lived for two years in Haiti and had been exposed to severe poverty there. But the numbers and concentration of poverty in this Indian city of 13 million were on a different order of magnitude.

On a Sunday morning, as Marilyn and I were walking to church, we came upon a man hunkered down along the road; he appeared to be very sick. I noticed his pallor and swollen hands and feet. I tried to talk to him, but he didn't seem to hear. We had only been in India for several weeks, and I didn't know what social services were available. I put some rupees in his shirt pocket and walked on, feeling like the priest who left the man by the side of the road in the story of the Good Samaritan in the Bible. When I came home from church, the man was gone. I never found out what happened to him.

Later I talked to some of my Indian friends and colleagues. Their responses ran the gamut from "Get used to it, this is Calcutta" to "You can't be all things to all people" to "Once you start helping, you'll never stop—and you have *your* life too." Some middle- and upper-class Indians who had grown up in Calcutta were so accustomed to these street scenes that they literally didn't see the poverty and the desperate situations of the multitudes of people around them.

I came to the realization that I would need to find a way to deal with the poverty and the pain—and my reactions to these realities. If I didn't, I would lose my ability to do the work that was the reason Marilyn and I went to India in the first place. I knew I couldn't allow myself to get too emotionally involved on a daily basis. At the same time, I felt strongly that if I lost all compassion it would be time for me to go home. The image that came to me was the need to "compartmentalize" my feelings—to place them on hold in order to make the necessary management decisions in my role as director of the area development program. By finding this kind of balance between the competing polarities of *too much* and *too little* emotional involvement, I subsequently was able to stay in India for seven enjoyable and fruitful years.

CHAPTER FOURTEEN

Even-Keeled:
Consistent and Dependable

My friend Lynn (see Chapter 4) builds wooden boats. When he starts to build, the first task is to lay the keel. A sturdy beam that runs from bow to stem, the keel is the foundation or spine that gives strength to the body of the boat. In one craft, Lynn poured 700 pounds of molten lead to form the keel and give the boat extra stability when the seas got rough. When large ships are built, the importance of laying the keel may be observed by a special ceremony. A boat or ship that has a broken keel is usually written off as unfixable.

Many of us have heard the phrase *even-keeled*. When applied to a person, we mean this person is steady and consistent, not given to fits of anger, periods of morose depression or wide swings in emotion. The judgment and ways of relating by such individuals remain steady and generally predictable.

As a doctor, I was aware of the need to be even-keeled. I could not let emotions get in the way of the decisions I needed to make for my patients. It is asking a great deal of patients to place their trust in a doctor who has the power to make life-and-death decisions. This is comparable to the trust that a passenger getting on an airplane places in the pilot or an astronaut places in the competence of the people who prepare and control the spaceship. This kind of trust requires the perception of virtual infallibility—no mistakes (at least no serious ones). It takes even-keeled individuals to earn that kind of trust.

Early in my medical practice, I knew I needed to gain the trust of my patients. As with all young doctors, relating to patients had always been with the looming presence of an experienced mentor at my side or in the background. Now I was asking patients to trust *me.*

Two levels of trust

With time, I learned that patients had two levels of trust. First, they wanted to know if I was competent. Did I know enough to take care of their medical problems? Was I keeping up with the latest in medical advances, knowing that some of what I learned in medical school was rapidly becoming obsolete? I discovered that most patients were ready to give the doctor the benefit of any doubt and assume that he or she *knew.* Within the first weeks of practice, one of the older surgeons said ruefully, "When I started practice, patients demanded doctors with experience. Now that I am old and have the experience, patients want the young doctors because they have the latest information."

Second, patients wanted to know if I *cared*. They wondered, *Would this young doc care for me as a unique individual? Would he care about my feelings and not just whether I had arthritis or high blood pressure?* I learned that caring for patients' feelings meant that I would be nonjudgmental and respectful. One day a young mother brought her 3-week-old baby to me. She asked if she should be using the drops from the hospital on her son's circumcision or belly button. At the time of discharge from the hospital she was given a complimentary bottle of vitamin drops "to be given to the baby by mouth." Apparently she hadn't read this directive. Caring for this young mother meant that I repressed my urge to laugh. Instead, I simply told her she could stop using the drops now.

The importance of respect

I became aware that respect for patients meant respect for *all* patients. A man who was very drunk came to the emergency room after an accident. He was agitated, kicking and swearing at those of us who needed to examine him for the extent of his injuries. In that situation, there is a natural tendency to respond in kind—roughly and with irritation. In my mind, it came to me strongly that even in his belligerent drunken state, the man was a person created in the image of God, deserving of respect and dignity.

'I became aware that respect
for patients meant respect
for *all* patients.'

As a physician, I also needed to extend respect to my colleagues and to other medical personnel. As medical director of a small hospital later in my professional life, I found that respect made all situations easier. I began to hear stories of the disruptive behavior of one of the doctors on the staff. Nurses and patients alike told stories of his anger over trivial things. I sent him a note asking that he stop in to see me the next Monday. He stopped by on Friday saying he didn't want to delay the matter over the weekend. I told this dignified doctor in his mid-60s what I was hearing and asked, "What is going on?" He replied, "I just get so damn mad ... I can't help myself, and I tell people off." Without any statement of judgment, I asked him what he thought should be done. He said, "I think I need to retire." We then talked about when he could retire so that there would be time for a replacement to be found. As he was leaving, he shook my hand and said (with tears in his eyes), "Thank you for being so kind to me." His attitude and performance were exemplary over the next six months until he retired.

The even-keeled doctor will be consistent, steady and focused. In my growing-up years, sometimes with nine children in one room of the house, there was a constant hubbub. I had the reputation among my siblings of being able to continue to read a book "when the house was falling down." This kind of focus carried through to my life as a doctor. I had to turn off any noises in my head that clamored for attention. I couldn't waver in my attention to patients when the weather turned sour, or when I had an argument with my wife, or when I just didn't feel top-notch. Through it all, I needed to maintain my equilibrium and a cool demeanor.

Another example: A patient came to see me very discouraged and disheartened. She had been ill for weeks with vague symptoms. Her regular doctor did a number of tests to try to come up with a diagnosis. When the tests were complete, he told her that all the tests were negative—and in reporting that fact he assumed she would feel relief that she didn't have the dread diseases they had tested for. Her doctor implied that her symptoms were "in your head" and discharged her without a return appointment. Her symptoms continued, and she felt abandoned by her physician who didn't recognize her need for continued support and a solution to her problem. I came to realize the need to be consistently persistent.

I also had to work to develop a sense of calmness and equanimity in relation to my emotions. A cardiac arrest is one of the most critical medical crises. This is the time for urgent action. It is not a time for leadership by committee. The person leading the resuscitation sets the tone for this emergency. If the person in charge is calm and decisive, this will quickly be imparted to the other members of the team. I recall working with a team of experienced nurses to resuscitate a patient who had a cardiac arrest. Afterward, someone noted that we had been so focused that we had been *whispering* our directions to each other during the resuscitation, something none of us could recall happening before during a cardiac arrest. Calm and focused leadership had made everyone more efficient and able to concentrate on the complicated task of restarting a heart that had stopped.

'Heal thyself' ... 'know thyself'

Ultimately, if doctors are to serve their patients well, they must follow the admonition of Jesus in the fourth chapter of the Book of Luke in the Bible: "Physician, heal thyself." Luke himself was a doctor, so it's not surprising that he quoted Jesus in this regard. For me in my medical career, this insight has had a number of dimensions:

- **Accountability.** There were days when I had to consciously clear my mind of distractions and preoccupations so that I could give my full attention and best effort to every patient encounter. I needed to be consistently accountable to patients, day after day.
- **Humility.** This quality drives one to always get better, to be committed to life-long learning, to absorb new information and to learn from patients and sometimes painful experience.
- **Recognize cultural differences.** I needed to recognize my own cultural background that shaped my patterns of communication, customs and beliefs—and be sensitive to patients from different (sometimes strikingly different) cultural or ethnic backgrounds. To be effective, I needed to be aware of these differences, to be nonjudgmental and to find ways to bridge the cultural gaps.

- **Face the ultimate reality of one's own death.** This reality hit me the most forcefully, not when a patient died, but when a young man I recruited to work as director of respiratory therapy was suddenly killed with his wife and infant child in a car accident. Through that experience and facing the reality of my own death (when I had a heart attack in India in 1996), I have become better able to walk with patients in their own end-of-life journey.
- **A balance of empathy and objectivity.** Empathy will lead the caregiver to understand more than the science-based part of medical practice, to appreciate the social and psychological factors that affect the patient. On the other hand, the ability to be objective is essential to making decisions based on logical reasoning. I talk more abut this in the chapter on compassion.
- **A variety of roles to play.** As a primary care physician, I needed to assume vastly different roles: to be the stern disciplinarian to the undisciplined, to be a compassionate listener to the grieving, to encourage the discouraged, to be a source of hope for those in despair.

'There's a healthy balance between introspective reflection and confident action.'

Not only did the Greek philosopher Socrates famously utter the dictum "Know thyself," he also said, "The unexamined life is not worth living." Healthcare workers (and all of us) must find the time to lean back in our chairs and ask what this is all about. For me, doing this helps to better see things in perspective and to see connections between things that might otherwise seem to be random events. This kind of self-scrutiny takes discipline and a belief that the precious time spent doing it is worth it. I spoke above about the balance between empathy and objectivity. There's also a healthy balance between introspective reflection and confident action.

Just as a captain guides his ship safely past rocky shoals or just as a pilot safely lands his plane in a storm, a doctor points the way for patients past the rough physical and emotional places to better health. To earn the trust of those for whom the doctor is responsible requires a steady hand at the tiller and an even-keeled temperament, both of which are essential, day in and day out.

CHAPTER FIFTEEN

Drifting—or a Life of Purpose

Early in our marriage, Marilyn and I made a conscious decision that we needed to take charge and become more proactive in the way we lived. This meant making both the smaller
and larger decisions with a view to the overall purpose of our
lives.

In 1971, after six years of family practice, we left our home
in west-central Ohio and went to Columbus to further my
medical education. We had lived in Bellefontaine, a modestly
sized town, where we were raising our four children. I came
to believe that I could serve our community and my own
interests better in medicine with further training in internal
medicine.

When we returned to Bellefontaine in 1973, Marilyn and I
decided we needed a garage for our home in the country. An
architect surveyed our three acres and returned with his pro-
posal. He laid out plans to change our driveway and build a
garage. Then he offered added options: a family room with a
portico over the new driveway, a swimming pool behind the
garage and a tennis court beside the pool. Oh, and how about
a golf green at the other end of the three-acre property?

We looked at the plans and projected the price tag. We
decided we could afford the cost, but the project would take
a significant amount of our available money for many years
to come. This would limit our options for any future change
of plans. We decided to move the driveway and build the

garage. Swimming and tennis courts were available only two miles from our home, and we saw no need for them. The golf green? There were courses in the area. I remember celebrating that we had been able to define our needs versus our wants.

Charting the next phase of our lives

In 1982 Marilyn and I enrolled our youngest daughter in college and took off for a week of bicycling in New Hampshire. We went with specific agenda—that having spent 25 years raising our children, we now wanted to discuss what to do the next 25 years. We decided three things: (1) In five years we wanted to be in a different place doing something different, (2) we wanted to be in place of service where we would both have assignments, and (3) we wanted the next assignment to build on our previous training and experiences.

Seven years later (yes, we missed our target by a couple of years) we found a situation that met all of our criteria. In 1989 we agreed to a four-year contract with Mennonite Central Committee, an international relief and development agency, to lead its program in India. These assignments were as volunteers on a volunteer salary—a salary cut from six figures to about $260 a month. We stayed in India for seven years.

Several medical colleagues in the States questioned my sanity, pointing out that professionally I was at the height of my prestige and earning potential. Other people wondered if our motivation stemmed from our earlier experience in Haiti and a feeling of guilt about our position of relative wealth compared with the poor of the world. But the most common reaction from both colleagues and non-medical people was a wistful "I wish I could do that." When we talked about why they couldn't do something similar, it always seemed to be due to their financial obligations tying them to their present lifestyle.

One such person was my financial adviser. We talked about the need to control one's spending in order to allow some flexibility in choices later in life. A year later, he told me that, before our discussion, he and his wife were planning to move to a bigger house in a more prestigious neighborhood. Then they looked at where they were and realized that their house was adequate with a big lawn and neighbors who were their close friends. They knew that if they moved to a new house, they would lose their friends, so they stayed in the same house.

'We were committed to living
our lives intentionally,
making conscious decisions
rather than following
the course of least resistance.'

We were reminded that our decision about the swimming pool, the tennis court and the golf green gave us the freedom to leave my relatively lucrative medical practice and go to India. By now, we were committed to living our lives intentionally, making conscious decisions rather than following the course of least resistance.

At home in Calcutta

India and specifically Calcutta became our home, as noted, for seven years. We enjoyed our work and our associations.

Marilyn and I provided team leadership to the MCC work; I did very little medical work. Calcutta has few U.S. citizens, and most of our social life revolved around Indian friends. As part of our work, we traveled through much of India and were continually fascinated by its color and cultural diversity. Travel in India is always an adventure. The overnight train trips were physically strenuous and invariably fascinating. I found it difficult to sleep on the train and welcomed the calls of the tea *wallah* (servant) that indicated morning was approaching. Upon our return to Calcutta after a trip to the interior of India, it was a welcome sight to see our driver who took us to our humble but comfortable home.

Most Friday evenings, after the office closed, we risked dings and dents to our car as we maneuvered through the dense traffic—buses, trucks, hand-pulled rickshaws, motorcycles, bicycles, people walking, even the occasional cow—to a five-star hotel where we spent an hour relaxing (at our own expense). The hotel was truly an oasis of serenity from the clamor and hubbub of the streets outside. We got copies of the most recent *USA Today* and *International Herald Tribune* and drank our iced coffee. We absorbed the news of the world outside. I learned that the scores of the games of my favorite sports teams did not change even if I got the news five days late. At the end of each week Marilyn and I had the satisfaction that we had made a difference. Some positive things were happening that almost certainly would not have taken place had we not been there.

An unexpected personal crisis

Toward the end of our time in India, in 1996, I had a heart attack. For more than a year before, I'd had vague symptoms, including extraordinary tiredness while paying tennis. On a visit to the States in 1995 I had undergone a number of tests that seemed to rule out any impending heart trouble. In March 1996 we were at a tennis/golf club for several days in a belated celebration of our 40th wedding anniversary.

I got up early in the morning to play tennis with three acquaintances: two Indians and a Russian. After playing one set, I became excessively fatigued and, to the good-natured ribbing from my playing partners about getting old, I asked to sit for a breather. When the tiredness persisted, I told them I needed to quit the game. By the time I reached our room, I knew the problem was serious and probably a heart attack.

Marilyn contacted the hotel front desk and learned that there was a doctor on call for emergencies. It turned out to be a pediatrician. I was careful to describe my symptoms as a textbook description of a heart attack, and the doctor made arrangements for me to be admitted directly to a cardiac care unit in the best hospital in Calcutta. We called a taxi that took me to the hospital where I received good and modern care—blood tests and cardiograms that confirmed a significant heart attack.

As I was dozing off the first night in the hospital, I unexpectedly found myself praying the childhood prayer:

> *Now I lay me down to sleep,*
> *I pray the Lord my soul to keep,*
> *If I should die before I wake ...*

And I stopped short. I thought I *could* die before I wake. My next thought was that I didn't have a lot unfinished agenda with other people, so from that standpoint it would be all right if I died in my sleep that night. The next morning I remembered my last thought before sleeping, and it came to me forcefully that my family would be very sad if I died. I suddenly knew I had to live.

That first night after the heart attack I had a vivid dream. In my dream I was in a large room in the hold near the front of a ship. I noticed a red door where the ship came to a point. The door swung open and, when I saw the water surging forward, I could tell that the ship was backing away. It occurred to me that if I wanted to get off the ship, I needed to jump to the wharf. I jumped. That was the end of the dream.

'I almost certainly would not have survived had I been in a small village when the heart attack occurred.'

The next morning I remembered the dream in great detail, including the distinct grain of the wood on the wharf. The doctors told me that, during the night, my heart rate had dropped to a dangerously low 33 beats a minute. There's no way to definitely say that the dream was at the exact time my heart slowed. However, I recalled that three weeks earlier I had been traveling to small villages in the interior of India, at least 36 hours away from any advanced medical care. I almost certainly would not have survived had I been there when the attack occurred.

Living with purpose

On reflection, I felt that this sequence of events indicated that there was yet purpose for me to continue living. That belief has guided me since, and I continue to have a mild sense of urgency that there is work yet to do.

Since that experience, I get up each morning with a sense of gratefulness. I am convinced that out of gratefulness comes joy. This kind of joy has little to do with everyday circumstances. This attitude of gratefulness and joy was re-enforced by the people of Calcutta, which has been called "The City of Joy" by Dominique Lapierre in his book by the same name. Their joy comes from gratefulness for the little things that come along. There is no sense of entitlement—of deserving things because of who they are—but rather a sense of gratitude for the good things that happen, like knowing where their next meal is coming from.

Elie Wiesel, a survivor of the Nazi Holocaust, was told a decade after World War II that he had survived so that he could write the story for those who died. He said that, having survived, he feels he needs to give meaning to his survival. In a real sense that is what we all need to do: give meaning to why we are given a few days—or many—here on earth.

CHAPTER SIXTEEN

Mother Teresa and Other Inspiring
Models of Dedication

Over the years, it has been my good fortune to come to know
many people whose lives have inspired me and became mod-
els for me. In the following pages I profile three individuals
who shared humility and the willingness to give up comfort
and possible prosperity to work for the welfare of those who
are less fortunate. They all have a strong sense of justice and
the will to do something about the *in*justices they see around
them. This sense of justice comes from a deep love of people
and is driven by strongly held religious faith and beliefs.

Mother Teresa

In 1996 I was hospitalized in Calcutta with a heart attack. A
get-well card from Mother Teresa was among the many well-
wishes I received. Mother Teresa's card was the familiar picture of Jesus carrying a lamb, surrounded by a flock of sheep.
The card had a hole and an imprint that told me it had been
thumb-tacked to a board. On the lamb in Jesus' arms, Mother
had written the word "you." On the back side of the card she
wrote:

> *Dear Dr. Glen E. Miller*
> *Be the little lamb in the arms of Jesus who loves you.*
> *I will pray for you [to] get well soon.*
> *God bless you,*
> *M. Teresa, MC*

I had first come to know Mother Teresa and the Missionaries of Charity four years earlier. At the time of my heart attack, Mother Teresa was the leader of more than 3,000 Missionaries of Charity working in at least 100 countries. In the course of her work, she related to thousands of people. A visitor asked Mother how she could minister to so many people. Her disarmingly simple answer was, "One at a time." With the get-well card she sent to me, I had become one of those one-at-a-time people whom Mother encouraged and blessed.

I never particularly hankered to meet famous people. Famous people, after all, never seemed to want to meet *me,* and when I was in a line to greet one of them, it was obvious that techniques were in play to move people along and not take too much of the great person's time. So, even though I lived in Calcutta, the home of Mother Teresa, for a couple of years I did not seek the means to meet her.

The opportunity to meet Mother Teresa came on the occasion of the 50-year celebration of our organization (Mennonite Central Committee) being established in India. Mother agreed to be the keynote speaker for this auspicious occasion. She arrived on time and after introductions, we sat together, waiting for the festivities to start. However, the welcome flower leis were late in arriving. During this delay, Mother and I sat in the front row of the seats in the *shamiana* (tent-like structure) as guests filed in behind us.

'Mother Teresa and I sat in the front row as guests filed in behind us; for 30 minutes we talked.'

For 30 minutes we talked. (Her English was excellent.) I learned that the Missionaries of Charity had started in Calcutta about four years after the 1942 arrival of MCC. Mother told me of her former life as a cloistered teaching nun inside the walls of St. Loretta School—one of the elite girls schools in Calcutta. On September 10, 1946, at the age of 36, on her way to the hill station for her annual retreat, she passed through the streets of Calcutta. On the train ride north, she said Jesus called her to leave the shelter of the school walls and go into the streets of Calcutta to work among the poor people. During our conversation a number of people came to greet her and to seek her blessing.

Later I got to know Mother for her compassion, her focus on helping the poorest of the poor and for her love of Jesus. In December 1992 a Hindu mob destroyed a Muslim mosque that had been claimed several centuries before as a sacred place for Hindus. This act stirred passions all over India. Nightly the newscasts gave running totals of the number of people killed in rioting throughout all of North India.

There was an absolute curfew that allowed no movement in the streets of Calcutta. However, the *Calcutta Telegraph* said that Mother Teresa was traveling the streets trying to help bring calm. In the middle of the week she issued an appeal for peace that was widely credited with bringing the violence under control. In the newspaper she said in part …

> *… We are all God's children—and we have been created … to love and be loved. God loves each one of us with an everlasting live—we are precious to Him. Therefore nothing should separate us … Religion is a gift of God and is meant to help us to be one heart full of love. God is our Father—and we are all his*

children—we are all brothers and sisters. Let there be no distinctions of race or colour or creed.

Let us not use religion to divide us. In all the Holy Books, we see how God calls us to love. Whatever we do to each other—we do to Him because he has said, "Whatever you do to the least of my brothers, you do it to Me." Religion is a work of love—it must unite us. It should not destroy peace and unity.

Works of love are works of peace—to love we must know one another. Today, if we have no peace, it is because we have forgotten that we are all God's children. That man, that woman, that child is my brother and sister. If everyone could see the image of God in his neighbour, do you think we would still have such destruction and suffering? ...

So, please, please, I beg you in the name of God, stop bringing violence, destruction and death to each other, and especially to the poor who are always the first victims.

Let us remember that the fruit of religions is to bring the joy of loving through the joy of sharing.[8]

After the curfew was lifted, I went to see Mother with the offer of cooking oil and wheat flour for the poor and home-less, knowing that she would be in touch with the people who were burned out of their homes and most in need. I asked her about traveling the roads during the curfew when the soldiers had orders to shoot to kill "anything that moves." With a smile, she told me about going to trouble spots in the city with only her driver. She said, "I sat in the front seat with the driver and when we came to a road block, the soldiers would stop us, but I just raised my head [Mother had become stoop-shouldered as she got older], and the soldiers would wave us through."

Mother Teresa was venerated by people of all walks of life—the old and the young, the poor and the rich, Christian, Hindu and Muslim. Each day that she was in town she received visitors on the small second-floor walkway between her living quarters and the Mother House Chapel. Usually five to twenty people waited their turn to see her. The sister who organized these times always asked me to wait until the others had been seen so that Mother would have more time for me.

As I waited, I watched Mother greet her visitors. Each person got Mother's full attention. Most asked for her blessing. A Hindu family caught my attention—mother, father and 2-year-old girl. The child was adopted from the Missionaries of Charity Orphanage and was now coming to visit Mother on her second birthday. When it came their turn to see Mother, the girl threw herself down at Mother's feet and kissed her feet in the classical Bengali style as her parents beamed.

One day Mother told us about her early days of the Missionaries of Charity. She said she was teaching some street children by writing letters in the dust with a stick. She noticed that one child looked sick. When she asked him, he said he hadn't had anything to eat for three days. Mother gathered rice and *dal* (lentils) and took it to his home. Immediately, the boy's mother divided the food into two portions. When Mother Teresa asked this Hindu mother what she was doing, she replied that her Muslim neighbors had had nothing to eat for four days, and half the food would go to them.

Mother Teresa and her work among the poor in Calcutta became known to the world after she was awarded the Nobel Peace Prize in 1979. I was aware that what Mother did was national and international news. One Saturday morning we had an appointment at the Mother House with her and were apologetically told that Mother was not there; she had been called to meet with the prime minister of Vietnam.

Each year Mother observed her birthday with a celebratory mass. As invited guests, we often sat close to her, sometimes making the national telecasts as a result. When it came time to receive the sacraments, we as non-Catholics were not invited to participate. I sensed that Mother regretted that.

'Mother told her kindly, "Go home and find your own Calcutta."'

The Missionaries of Charity had many visitors who worked in their various programs. One of these visitors expressed the desire to stay there long term and work. Mother told her kindly, "Go home and find your own Calcutta."

There may be a tendency to view Mother Teresa as other-worldly or as a saint (indeed, she appears to be on the Roman Catholic "track" to sainthood as this book is written). While I was always impressed with her single-mindedness in help-ing the poor, motivated by her love of Jesus, every time I saw her I was impressed with her humanity and the epitome of what a human being can be. Her humanity came through in constantly being attuned to the moment even though there must have been a multitude of matters pressing on her. I also found her playful sense of humor endearing and even charmingly self-deprecating.

She died in September 1997 (at the age of 87), just a few months after we had left India upon completing our seven-year assignment. I regret that I could not attend the funeral of this remarkable woman, one I counted as a friend. Some of our MCC colleagues in India were able to attend.

The day after Mother Teresa's death Marilyn and I were on a speaking trip in Ontario, and I showed the audience the card that Mother had sent me the year before. Afterward a woman who had grown up Catholic came up to me and asked, "Could I touch that card?" Such was the veneration and esteem in which Mother Teresa was held around the world.

Dr. Joyce Siromoni

I first met Dr. Joyce Siromoni in 1992 when I, along with some of my MCC development staff, went to visit her and see the work she was doing. After traveling through block after block of congested Calcutta, we arrived at Paripurnata. Joyce greeted me with a broad smile of welcome.

As we entered the building, I noted that it was small and clean. Joyce introduced us to her staff of five or six social workers and other staff members. I immediately wondered where there was space for all these people to work. She also introduced us to some of the eight women they were serving. These women had a history of mental illness.

Joyce was born in what is now Pakistan. Her family later moved to India where her father worked as a homeopathic doctor, frequently treating patients without charge. She went to school in a Christian boarding school. At a young age, after visiting her doctor aunt, she announced, "I will become a doctor one day." Years later she graduated from Vellore Christian Medical College and fulfilled that prediction.

Joyce married Paul, an industrial management consultant. Joyce worked in various rural clinics with women's medicine. While living in Bangalore, she became aware of the needs of mentally ill people and took several into her home for months at a time. She realized the value of a "therapeutic community"—of surrounding the afflicted person with loving, non-judgmental people. Later, living in Calcutta, she invited a young homeless drug addict to live in her home. He later became a successful journalist.

In 1990 Joyce read an article in the newspaper titled "800 NCLs Languishing in Jails in West Bengal." The legal name for the mentally ill was non-criminal lunatics. The article stated that these women, confused and disoriented, were taken off the streets "for their own protection" and so that "no harm will come to the public." The women were living under deplorable conditions: often naked, without toilet facilities and sometimes chained. Some of the women had been in jail for more than eight years.

Joyce began to look for like-minded people to address the desperate needs of these women. With the help of Justice Mahitosh Majumdar and other people she formed Paripurnata, which means "hope for wholeness" in Hindi. Joyce described the mission of Paripurnata as extending "unconditional love that is full of grace, patience and kindness, does not talk ill of others but in love upholds all people to God." As we were touring the house, Joyce told us of her vision for a larger building some day to serve more women in these circumstances. In 2002 we returned to Calcutta and visited Joyce; she proudly showed us the new building with room for 25 women. She also told us of the extensive outpatient clinics under their direction that continue to serve former residents of Paripurnata and provide mental health services to other members of the community.

I asked Joyce for stories of several women who had been rehabilitated. She told me the story of "Sushmita" who was released from jail to their care. She lived with them at Paripurnata for six months where she learned to sew, took her medicine regularly and re-learned the skills to live in society. The social workers tried to find her family, but after eight years in deplorable conditions Sushmita remembered few details. The staff followed one lead to a small village where they hoped to find Sushmita's sister. For an hour they talked with a woman there, but there was no recognition on the part of either person. As they were turning to leave, the village woman asked Sushmita where she got the bracelet on her ankle. She answered that her father had given it to her. The village woman said, "You are my sister." Recognition broke through like the morning sun. A joyful and tearful reunion ensued.

Joyce writes about another woman:

Lily was 52 years when she came to Paripurnata for psycho-social rehabilitation. She has been suffering from schizophrenia. Her husband admitted her to Calcutta Mental Hospital 8 years ago. He visited her once a year during Puja Festivals, taking food and clothes. He got married while she was in the hospital and had a son by the second lady.

While Lily was undergoing rehabilitation at Paripurnata, we contacted her husband. He is a good man but refused to take her back. One day she asked him, "I am your legal wife. You married me, don't you think that you should also help me? I will not interfere in your family life or with your second wife and son, but you owe me some help so that I too can live."

This made the husband think and he agreed to help her after she was discharged.

He helped to find a room and paid the rent and also Rs. 200/- every month for living expenses. Paripurnata helped her to set up her home with cooking vessels and stove. She worked as domestic help and gradually raised her income from Rs. 40/- to Rs. 1200/ per month by working in 3 or 4 houses.

About 2 years ago, the house owner pressured her to leave the house. She assured the landlord that as soon as she found another accommodation she would leave. One day, when she was gone, the house-owner locked her house. She straight away walked off to the police station and brought the police. The police asked the house owner if Lily was paying the rent. She said, "Yes, up to date." The police asked her to open the lock, and not to disturb her, till she gets another house. This is EMPOWERMENT!!

About the same time, the second wife died and Lily's husband fell sick. Lily went every week to see him and take some fruit for him.

115

I [Joyce] asked her, "Lily your husband left you in the mental hospital for 8 years, and yet you take fruit for him." She laughed and said, "After all he is support- ing me by giving financial help. I should do some- thing for him, especially when he is not well."

This I would say is LOVE. She never forced herself to stay with him and maintained her dignity, but showed responsibility and dignity to care for him when he was not well.

Joyce and the stories of women's lives literally redeemed from a human waste heap helped to clarify my thinking on right and wrong and good and evil. It seems to me that we do wrong when we deny or hinder any person from reaching toward his or her God-given potential. We do good when we are part of helping persons become whole and move toward what God intends for them. This message may be summed up by the motto of Paripurnata: *"Unconditional love has great healing power."*

Dr. Willard Krabill

In the last four and a half years, Willard became a close friend and confidant. We played golf together about every week for six to seven months a year. In the off months, we regularly had breakfast together.

I write this three days after Willard died on January 16, 2009. The diagnosis of cancer was made only six months earlier. The morning of the day before he died, I woke up with a strong feeling that I should go to see Willard. I had been stop- ping in to see him about once a week, occasionally more often. I hadn't seen him for more than a week because he was unresponsive, and I thought he wouldn't recognize me. But on this morning, I felt that even in his present state, there might be a sliver of consciousness, so that he would hear me if I went to say goodbye. I also felt that going to see him was the right thing to do, even if he didn't or couldn't respond.

> 'I felt that going to see him
> was the right thing to do,
> even if he didn't
> or couldn't respond.'

When I got there, Willard recognized me and mouthed, "Thank you for coming." When I held his hand in mine he squeezed my hand and held on. I told him I had come to say goodbye and thanked him for what he meant to me—that he was an inspiration to me. I told Willard that he had taught me how to strive for perfection.[9] I also thanked him for all the good times we had and our discussions that knew no boundaries. With my face close to his, I said to Willard, "Go in peace, God will take care of you." He died the next morning.

Willard had admitted to being a perfectionist. When we played golf, each of us could visualize the perfect shot: its trajectory and where the ball should land. Willard had a standard response when the ball sliced off at an angle or became a "grass cutter" that hugged the ground. He would say in his quiet voice, "Not exactly." But I never saw him get frustrated with a bad shot.

Not exactly. Using that phrase told me that Willard knew what "exactly" was. Just as he knew the perfect golf shot, he knew the right way to do things in his personal relationships and professional life. He was persistent in his concern for justice and morally correct ways to do things. It is clear that his strong sense of justice came from a loving concern for all people. He had a way of accomplishing great things, without offending, through his gentle, yet persistent, approach; his soft-spokenness; and his ability to communicate a clear message. In my mind, Willard stood tall. Not until several months after the diagnosis of cancer did it occur to me that he was of small stature.

Willard told me that early in life his father had advised him, "Don't follow where the path leads. Go where there is no path and make a trail." Willard followed that advice and became a national leader in advocating for the presence of fathers in the delivery room at the time of the birth of their child. He was a constant learner, with postgraduate training in obstetrics, public health and medical ethics. He worked for 24 years as a professor at Goshen College where he created an innovative healthcare plan for employees, with emphasis on prevention, and taught classes in human sexuality that highlighted, for a generation of students, the holistic nature of sexuality. This class became the best-attended course on campus. Willard greatly appreciated his former students, several of whom participated in his care over the last months of his life.

We continued to play golf for about three months after the diagnosis of incurable cancer. I told him I was available to play whenever he wanted. We golfed for the last time in the early fall. The day was sunny and warm. Willard noted that this was probably the last time he could play. It was such an enjoyable time, and that day he repeatedly said how much he relished being outdoors on such a lovely day.

I miss Willard. He was a major touchstone that gave balance to my life. He inspired me by his faith walk and the consistency of his wanting to follow the way of Jesus. Willard is gone from my sight but not from my memories. I am left with a deep sense of gratitude that Willard Krabill was part of my life the last 4½ years.

CHAPTER SEVENTEEN

Preparing to Die Well

"Charley." That's what his friends and relatives called him. He was my father. At age 85, he made one of the most important decisions of his life. Over the span of years his choices had been informed by his strong identity as a Mennonite and by the community in which he lived. His decisions gave direction to the way that the lives of his nine children unfolded. In a time of economic depression he was the stabilizing pillar who kept food on the table and made the payments on our 80-acre farm. As retirement approached, he with my mother chose to continue to invest their lives in others by engaging for six years in voluntary service programs in Mississippi, Florida and Puerto Rico.

At age 65, Charley had developed diabetes. In the ensuing years as he aged, I tried to talk to him on three separate occasions about how much medical care he wanted and what limitations should be placed. Each time, he politely turned the conversation aside. He clearly was not ready to talk about it.

Twenty years after the onset of diabetes, Charley was hospitalized in failing health. His doctor told him his kidneys were failing and he needed to consider dialysis. He gathered the family, and together they faced the decision whether to allow the kidney disease to progress—or to start dialysis and prolong his life (Marilyn and I were in India at the time). He asked the assembled family members what they thought. Each of them in turn said they felt it really was his decision. The family prayed together. After the prayer, Dad said, "I think I know the answer. I have had a good life. I outlived two wives. If Katherine [his second wife] were still living, I feel I would want dialysis, but I see no reason to prolong my life further."

'Clearing the way to the other side'

Charley's kidney failure gradually progressed. As the toxins in his blood accumulated, he had periods of mild confusion, but he never questioned his decision to forgo dialysis. On the evening before he died, he called his children together. His mind was remarkably clear. He went around the room in his wheelchair and asked each person for forgiveness for any wrong he had done. At his request, and in the Mennonite tradition, he was then anointed with oil, not for healing but, in his words, to "clear the way to the other side." At bedtime, when his nurse said, "I'll see you in the morning, Charley," he responded, "Oh no, I won't be here in the morning." He died peacefully at 5:30 a.m.

'Trust, respect and open communication among those involved in end-of-life decisions are the keys that will help navigate through these stressful times.'

Trust, respect and open communication among those involved in end-of-life decisions are the keys that will help navigate through these stressful times. Charley faced his decision about dialysis secure in the knowledge that his family wanted the best for him and confident that the support of his family and medical caregivers would remain strong. He also was confident that both his family and professional care-givers would honor his wishes with regard to further care, including the decision to forgo dialysis, knowing his life would thereby be shortened.

Charley was certain that his caregivers would do everything in their power to make his remaining days as comfortable as possible, with his dignity respected. And finally, he knew that his wishes about any limitations on the extent of medical care would be respected, including the right to say "enough" and request no further interventions that might prolong his life. Dad made these decisions while his mind was yet clear, knowing that if later he were unable to participate in making medical decisions he could have full confidence that those of us designated to make such decisions for him would follow his wishes because we had discussed the issues in detail.

Many religions view death as a passage to another (and better) life. Christians face death as a transition into a new life in the presence of God. With our families, we can make choices that ease that transition and lead to a "good death." That's what Charley had. That's what I want.

PART III

Further Exploration of Healthcare Issues

CHAPTER EIGHTEEN

Your Choice of a Primary Care Physician

It takes only a moment of reflection to realize the tremendous advances in healthcare over the last 50 (or even 10 to 20) years. Despite the wealth of information available on Internet and other sources, many people are confused or "lock up" when it comes to making healthcare decisions. Detailed instructions from a doctor may be completely forgotten or misunderstood. About half of Americans fail the "health literacy test."

In a nationwide study[10] a statistical analysis was done on the number of people who have a "usual source of care." Overall, 78% of people in the United States reported having a USC or a PCP (primary care physician). The percentage having a PCP varied according to age and ethnicity, with seniors at 94%; 18- to 24-year-olds, 65%; Hispanics, 60%; and non-Hispanics, 81%. As one would expect, there was a wide difference between the insured (83%) and uninsured (47%) with regard to having a PCP.

The data from this study support the reasons in favor of having a PCP. Patients with a usual source of care had:
- Better access to health services
- Better preventive services
- Fewer inappropriate emergency room visits
- Shorter length of stay in the hospital
- Better continuity of care
- Better health status

People without a PCP had poorer access to necessary health services and poorer health status. These factors were particularly evident in patients with chronic disease who lacked the continuity of care that a PCP would provide.

A major measure of an active collaboration between doctors and their patients is the degree to which patients feel they participate in the decisions regarding their healthcare. The study looked at the perceived degree of control that patients felt they had in making their healthcare decisions. Overall, 52% said they "always" participated in the decisions, with higher rates for high school graduates than non-graduates, insured than non-insured, Northeast than West residents and non-metropolitan than metropolitan residents.

The authors of the article conclude that there is need to improve the quality of patient/physician communication that will increase the participation of patients in their healthcare. This is particularly true of lower socioeconomic groups and in urban areas. For those persons who feel they have control over their healthcare decisions, education will help them to ask appropriate questions that will lead to better healthcare and improved health status.

Access to healthcare

The healthcare system is complex. A good working relationship with a PCP is a key entry point into the system. A PCP who is available for routine care of acute and chronic diseases is essential. Without a PCP there will be more likelihood of frustration, delay in treatment and increased cost. The probability of wrong turns in any diagnostic problem may well lead to delays and even life-threatening medical problems. When more complicated problems arise and specialized consultation is necessary, the PCP will be there to help the patient navigate through an often complicated system.

Preventive care

The PCP is necessary for an ongoing program of individualized preventive care. This program will include advice on healthy lifestyle choices and screening tests that catch diseases in their early stages. When chronic, longstanding problems arise, such as high blood pressure or diabetes, the PCP will provide the services that maintain control and prevent complications. In cases of rare diseases or complicated disease, a specialist will become the PCP.

Emergency care

A significant percentage of ER visits are inappropriate; there is no true emergency. When patients have a regular PCP who provides coverage for the hours when the office is closed, the need for most ER visits will be prevented. In cases of chronic diseases, the PCP will teach the patient how to control his or her disease, along with the symptoms that indicate the need for emergency treatment. One of the greatest benefits of a good relationship with a PCP is the peace of mind for the patient who knows exactly where he or she can go when medical care is needed.

Hospitalization

PCPs will know the capabilities of patients to provide care at home for themselves or their family members, as well as the social and economic factors that prevent being able to provide necessary care. The doctor can then with confidence expect that the patient will get the care he or she prescribes. This will both prevent hospitalizations and shorten hospital stays when they occur.

Continuity of care

The PCP knows past history of illnesses, surgeries, pertinent family history and social history. For example, if a young child has recurrent bronchitis, the doctor can address the issues in the home, such as smoking by one of the parents and the inhalation of secondhand smoke. A PCP can provide timely and appropriate care with less frustration and expense. It is essential that patients with chronic diseases have continuity of care so that there is common understanding between the patient and doctor about the goals of disease control that reduce complications and disability.

Health status

The end result of a working relationship with a PCP is improved health status. This connection will lead to less time lost from productive activity. Without a PCP, there is always the concern about where to go in the event of an emergency. For patients with chronic diseases and for parents with small children, the assurance of having an entry into the healthcare system and a caring doctor will bring peace of mind, as noted previously.

'For patients with chronic diseases
and for parents with small children,
the assurance of having an entry
into the healthcare system and a caring
doctor will bring peace of mind.'

The American College of Physicians in its recommendations for healthcare reform stresses the need for more PCPs, citing studies that show that communities where there are more PCPs there will be a 5% decrease in hospital admissions, fewer surgeries and fewer visits to the emergency room, all with savings in the cost of healthcare. The ACP also cites the need to provide incentives for young doctors to enter practice as PCPs. These incentives can include scholarships and a revamping of the methods of payment for services that reward PCPs more equitably in relation to medical specialists.

PCPs: Who are they?

There are now about 820,000 doctors in the United States. Thirty-seven percent of doctors (300,000) are PCPs, including family practitioners, general internists and pediatricians.

Each year 24,000 doctors enter the workforce. Of these new doctors, 16,000 have the M.D. (medical doctor) degree, and 3,000 have a D.O. (doctor of osteopathy) degree. In addition, about 5,000 IMGs (international medical graduates) enter medical practice. One in four doctors is female. The number of female doctors will continue to increase in this country since nearly half of entering medical school students are female, whereas most of the retiring doctors (such as the author) are male.

IMGs include individuals who emigrate from developing countries to the U.S. to improve their professional and personal lives. These medical school graduates need a visa to enter the U.S., must past a rigorous test to prove their basic knowledge and must have an appointment to an approved residency program. After completion of their medical training,

IMGs may stay in the U.S. if they go to a federally designated needy area and practice there for at least three years.

Among the IMGs there also are a number of U.S. citizens who have completed their medical school training in a foreign country. After their graduation they need an appointment to a residency program to fulfill their training requirements.

NPs (nurse practitioners) are nurses who have completed their RN (registered nurse) requirements and advanced training, usually leading to a master's degree and being credentialed by a national accrediting body. Their specialized training may be in one of a number of areas, such as adult or child care, anesthesia, critical care, midwifery and many others. In the area of primary healthcare, the NP functions independently to provide primary and preventive care under the overall supervision of a doctor. There are more than 120,000 NPs currently in practice. The American Nurses Association estimates that 60–80% of all primary and preventive care can be done by nurse practitioners.

What to look for in a PCP

One of my roles in our community and hospital was to orient new physicians. I invariably told then what one of my mentors had said to me, "Patients will generally assume that you *know,* but what they want to know is if you *care.*" Young doctors come out of years of training with their heads chock full of information. The physician enters his or her practice, and suddenly there is no mentor nearby. Then the doctor must apply that knowledge in consistent ways through good days and bad days, in times of elation and in times of discouragement. Despite all the personal peaks and valleys in life, the doctor must give the impression of calmness and equanimity.

In considering prospective doctors, one needs to ask two simple questions:
- Do they know, and do they care?
- Can I trust this doctor to make potentially the most important decisions in my life, and will he or she care enough to do that consistently?

In looking for healthcare providers, it's important to assess their communication skills. Does the PCP have the ability and patience to explain things to me so that I understand them? Is the doctor open to discussing the diagnosis and alternatives for treatment, or is he or she more inclined toward the parent-like role that prescribes without discussion? Does the doctor listen carefully without rushing to a diagnosis?

A central premise in this book is that the best quality of healthcare requires open communication between provider and consumer of healthcare where there is collaboration in making medical decisions. Some doctors don't see that as their role and tend to be impatient about time spent in discussion and explanation.

PCPs will place varying emphasis on preventive measures. As noted elsewhere, the U.S. healthcare system is more geared toward treating sickness than promoting health. In the search for a doctor, one needs to assess the stress placed on keeping well and maximizing health rather than just treating the present illness.

In selecting a doctor, you also will want to know the arrangements for medical care in the hours when the office is not open. Many doctors are in a group practice, and an assessment of the other partners in the group is important. A primary care doctor who doesn't provide any coverage during off hours but refers all calls to the emergency room is, in my view, a doctor to be avoided.

Persons with chronic illness, such as diabetes and high blood pressure, will want assurance that their new PCP has good experience in treating such diseases. As noted in an earlier chapter, good communication with your doctor will enable the patient and doctor to set goals of treatment and the means to reach those goals. Particularly in chronic cases, collaboration between the doctor and patient will keep the disease in check, help prevent complications and enhance the likelihood of leading a normal life.

> 'Good communication with your doctor
> will enable the patient and doctor
> to set goals of treatment and
> the means to reach those goals.'

There are, of course, other practical matters to look for in selecting a doctor, things that have no right or wrong answer. Would you prefer a man or woman doctor? Is the office located in a place convenient to you? Is the doctor affiliated with the hospital that you prefer? Does the doctor make hospital visits, or does he or she refer you to a hospital-based doctor?

What about a nurse practitioner for primary care? NPs are available in many doctors' offices and offer quality primary care. NPs often are able to spend more time with each patient, and most seek to be holistic in their approach, with an interest in health promotion and preventive measures. The choice of NP should be made on the same basis as the choice of a

PCP as described above, including competency, caring, communication and willingness to collaborate.

Getting connected with a PCP

There are several reasons why patients need to find a new doctor: moving to another community, a doctor moving or retiring, or the feeling that one's present doctor is not capable of meeting one's medical needs. This latter item may be due to a number of possibilities, but the most frequent is because of communication problems ("He doesn't listen to me"). And not uncommonly, the desire to change doctors is due to a perceived uncooperativeness on the part of the doctor's staff.

What are the steps in finding a new PCP? In what turned out to be a revealing exercise, I called three hospitals that serve nearly half a million people in my larger community and asked about finding a doctor. All three referred me to their Physician Referral Center. In one center I was given the name of a doctor who was accepting patients and advised to call and ask for an appointment. Staff persons in the physician's office would then decide if they would accept me as a patient. I asked why they would not accept me and was informed that it depended on the type of insurance I had. At one hospital only one doctor associated with the hospital would see patients on Medicaid.

At the other two hospitals I called, there was a list of doctors who were accepting patients. Persons without insurance or on Medicare or Medicaid are instructed to go to the emergency room if they have medical needs. If the ER staff determines that patients need follow-up, the ER will find a doctor for them. Clearly, individuals with health insurance have the inside track in getting in to see a doctor.

If you have insurance and are not in an HMO (health management organization), here are some practical suggestions about finding a new doctor:

1. Ask family, friends or co-workers for their suggestions. In this process, try to get a feel for how the doctor communicates. If you have special medical needs (such as chronic illness), ask about the doctor's experience in those areas.

2. Call the local Physician Referral Center; explain that you are a new patient and ask to be referred to a doctor. Someone there will give you the names of doctors accepting new patients.

3. Assess the doctor's training and experience. You can do this easily by clicking on *http://www.healthworldweb.com/pc/doctors/listing.* The website leads you through the process of finding doctors and nurse practitioners in a given location. You specify the language proficiency, location and specialty area of practice. Contact information is then available for each healthcare provider.

4. Check the location of the office, the doctor's hospital affiliation, training and board certification. (Board certification does not guarantee superior care, but it does indicate that the doctor has completed the training requirements to qualify for certification.)

5. If you have a chronic condition for which you are being treated, you may want to have as your PCP a doctor who specializes in this area. You can check the Directory of Medical Specialists at your local library.

6. Consider making an appointment with a staff member from the doctor's office to assure you of a match between your expectations and the way that healthcare is delivered in that office.

7. Before your first office visit, be sure to assemble your medical records, including your past medical history, drug allergies and current medications. If you have a chronic disease, take along recent test results used to monitor your medical condition.

A good working relationship with a primary care provider is essential to getting good healthcare. By taking the above steps, you will enhance your chances of finding a primary care physician who not only knows but cares!

CHAPTER NINETEEN

Prescription Drugs:
How to Bring Them Under Control

Are we becoming 'medicalized'?

In 1950 the most common drugs bought in this country were Geritol and Bayer aspirin. The pharmaceutical industry was minuscule compared with today. In 2002 Americans spent more than half of the total spent for prescription drugs in the world. The pharmaceutical industry through research and development of new drugs has added immeasurably to personal comfort and the human life span. Sociologists, however, wonder if too much emphasis is placed on relief of any discomfort—physical or emotional. The pressure is on pharmaceutical houses to produce yet more "miracle cures." Researchers work hard to develop new medicines to meet the demands. To some thoughtful observers, the sequence appears topsy-turvy—sometimes with the discovery of a new medicine that is "in search of a disease."

A report by the President's Council on Bioethics expressed concern that all of the problems of life tend to become *medical* problems and that "the pursuit of happiness and self-perfection would become part of the doctor's business."[11] The next logical step is that virtually all problems can be solved through the right medicines.

On her first appointment at my office Eileen brought along a shoebox full of bottles of pills—24 in all. She knew the names of all her medicines and what they were for—like the dear friends they had become. Seven of her medicines had apparently been prescribed for side effects of the other medicines. To put it mildly, I found it to be a challenge to wean Eileen off her medicines and address her ongoing hypochondriasis.

On any given day, you can hear the incessantly echoing exhortation on TV to "Ask your doctor" if this or that pill or prescription is right for you. Drug companies know that advertising is an effective way to promote their product—to get the patient to ask about (and create a desire for) the drug. In one U.S. study actors went to doctors complaining of symptoms of depression. A thorough examination would have revealed no evidence of depression in any of these actors, yet in 55% of office visits those actor-patients walked out with prescriptions for the mind-altering medicines they had asked for. It is noteworthy that only two countries in the world—the United States and New Zealand—permit prescription drug advertising on television.[12]

'On any given day, you can hear the incessantly echoing exhortation on TV to "Ask your doctor" if this or that pill or prescription is right for you.'

Representatives of the pharmaceutical industry add another dynamic to the promotion of the sale of drugs. These individuals represent the products of a single company and make their regular rounds to groups of doctors. Their function includes educating physicians on the benefits of newer medicines and checking with doctors or their office personnel about the need for samples. They drop off information on newer drugs or if possible meet with the doctor to inform him or her about the efficacies of new medicines. Their visits average about twice per month to each office. These drug reps have weekly updates on the prescribing patterns for each doctor for the medicines the company is currently promoting. In their visits they leave starter samples of their medicine. In some offices, the drug rep will arrange for lunch for the employees as often as once a week. Thankfully, the practice of gifts to the doctor and office staff is on the decline, and most doctors now routinely refuse them.

Drug reactions

Clearly, the growing availability of medicines over the last 100 years has brought comfort, delayed the ravages of chronic diseases and extended the lives of millions. However, the widespread use of medicines has its downside.

Adverse drug events (ADE) occur in about 1 in 20 hospitalizations in this country, accounting for billions (estimated $1.56 billion to $5.6 billion annually) of dollars in added costs and an average of 8 to 12 days of extended hospital stay.[13] According to one study, ADE caused permanent disability in 9.7% of cases. ADEs happen in the best of hospitals and include missed doses, improper administration technique, a doctor's order that was illegible, duplicate dosages, dangerous drug interactions, equipment failure, inadequate monitoring and preparations errors. Some of these problems have been addressed through computerized ordering and increased hospital pharmacist involvement in the process of drug administration.

It's impossible to predict who will have an ADE. There are no definable patient characteristics that can alert doctors to the likelihood of ADE. The type of medication also is not a predictor of ADE.

We constantly hear stories of a patient or family who questions the medicine being given and alertly prevents a medication error. It is recommended that all patients be aware of their medications and participate with the hospital staff—and one's doctor—in the correct administration.

> *One healthcare researcher, acquainted with these statistics, told me that if a member of his family is hospitalized, he or another member of the family will be in constant attendance with a notebook to record medications in an effort to prevent ADE.*

The high cost of research and development

Why do drugs cost so much? The up-front cost of a new drug is high, and the "road" is long to develop a new drug. There's an extensive process to get a drug approved for human use. Pharmaceutical companies go through multiple stages to gain approval of a drug. In the pre-clinical stages, testing is done on patients to prove that the drug is effective in the treatment of a condition or disease. At the same time the incidence of side effects—signs or symptoms that are undesirable—is measured. After testing on increasingly larger groups of patients, the drug company is ready to present the drug to the Food & Drug Administration (FDA) for approval.

According to a recent report from Tufts Center for Drug Development, the average cost of developing a new drug is $897 million. Only 22% of drugs under development eventually attain FDA approval. The stakes are high. Millions of dollars of investment in a new drug may end in failure if the drug is not effective or the incidence of side effects is so high that it isn't marketable. On the other hand, a successful drug that has wide usage can be the source of huge profits for the drug company. Kenneth Kaitin, director of the Tufts Center, observes that "drug development remains a time-consuming, risky and expensive process."

'A successful drug that has wide usage can be the source of huge profits for the drug company.'

The application process must state how the drug is manufactured and delineate how the body metabolizes the drug, its effectiveness, and incidence and severity of side effects. After all the information is submitted, the FDA may deny permission, require more testing or release the drug for human use. This decision is based on an assessment of the effectiveness and the safety of the drug. Follow-up monitoring of the drug for side effects also is required.

Despite high production costs, drug companies have enjoyed unprecedented profits over the last five years. The report, *Summary of Public Citizen: Congress Watch,* June 2002 (*http://www.citizen.org/documents/Pharma_Report.pdf*— accessed December 15, 2008) lists the following:

1. Drug company profits are higher than other 500 Fortune companies.
2. Drug prices rise faster than inflation.
3. Pharmaceutical companies are spending about twice as much for marketing and advertising as for research and development.

4. In 2002 drug companies had 675 paid lobbyists, seven for each U.S. senator.
5. Americans pay more for prescriptions than do the citizens of any other country in the world.

Occasionally a drug is thoroughly researched and developed to treat a specific disease, but on clinical trials it is found to be effective in treating another condition. Such was the case with Viagra, which initially was developed for treatment of high blood pressure and angina. Serendipitously, it was found to be effective in the treatment of male ED (erectile dysfunction). (One can only imagine how this discovery happened.) Viagra continues to have booming worldwide sales.

A case study: taxol

Taxol is an anti-cancer drug approved in 1992 for use in treating ovarian cancer and in 1994 for breast cancer. The latter is the most commonly diagnosed cancer (excluding skin cancer) among women, both in the United States and globally. As of 2005, it was estimated that 269,730 new cases of breast cancer would be diagnosed among women in this country.[14]

In 1960 the National Cancer Institute started a search for naturally appearing substances that may be effective against cancer. An extract from the Pacific yew tree was found to have strong anti-tumor activity. The Pacific yew tree is an endangered species and produces limited supplies of taxol. It would take six year-old trees to produce enough taxol to treat one patient. Ten years elapsed before further research into these properties was undertaken. Researchers were able to extract the active ingredient and identified its method of action of interfering with cell division. Various research centers began clinical trials, which were initially hampered by the lack of supply of naturally occurring taxol. In 1994, thirty-four years after the NCI began its search, the active ingredient was synthesized, and taxol became widely available for the treatment of breast cancer.

CHAPTER TWENTY

The Critical Need for Access to
Your Medical Records

In the last few years, Taiwan developed a model healthcare system that provides healthcare to all its citizens. This system was developed by healthcare experts after a two-year study of a number of healthcare systems around the world. The planners recognized that an essential ingredient in good healthcare was the ready availability of medical records. In the Taiwanese system, each patient has a plastic card with his or her pertinent medical information electronically imprinted. When a person visits a healthcare facility, the card is inserted into a reader and the healthcare provider instantly has access to the medical history. At the end of the visit, the results of the visit, including reports of laboratory tests and scans, are added to keep the record current.

Officials in Whatcom County in the state of Washington noted a few years ago that an estimated *one out of every seven hospital admissions could be prevented if the healthcare team had the medical records and that 20% of lab tests are repeated because lab reports are lost or not readily available.* The county has a website called the Shared Care Plan where residents of the county can register their medical history, including lab and surgery results. These results are stored online and available to anyone worldwide who has access to the Internet. The client participant has strict control over the content of the medical history and over who has access to the information. The service is free to residents of Whatcom County.

The county's website states:

> The Shared Care Plan is a self-management tool that will help you keep track of your health. Whether you are managing a chronic condition or are a fit athlete, the Shared Care Plan will help you manage your care. The information you enter online will be accessible to you and the people you specify from any Internet-ready computer around the world. Your Shared Care Plan can also be printed out as needed. Having this information with you when you visit your doctor may help you and your health care practitioners become partners in your care. *http://www.patientpowered. org/login.aspx* (accessed January 14, 2008).

Nationally, there is a movement toward electronic medical records. Currently just 7% of doctors use EMR in everyday patient care. Doctors are understandably reluctant to switch to EMR from systems that are tried and comfortable. The start-up costs are high, and the systems are not standardized. There is limited benefit to EMR if the system that the doctor uses in the office cannot "talk to" the hospital system or consulting doctors.

Until there is widespread use of EMR, individuals need to find a method that serves the purpose of making medical information available at the time of need, particularly in emergencies. It is critical that ER personnel know of severe allergies, chronic diseases, current medicines, and previous serious illnesses and surgeries.

> *A woman was brought to an emergency room after a car accident. The ER doctor did not know (and she was unable to tell him) about her severe allergic reactions to several medicines. She was given an injection*

of a medicine to which she was allergic. For the next two hours doctors had to fight to save her life from the severe allergic reaction. In the meantime, treatment of her injuries had to wait.

The need is for concise and pertinent information readily accessible at the time of an emergency. A medical history compiled *before* an emergency will obviously be more complete than trying to remember all relevant data at the time of an emergency.

'The need is for concise and pertinent information readily accessible at the time of an emergency.'

When seeing a new patient, doctors need the following information:
- **All new patients** should have:
    - A list of medicines, including over-the-counter meds
    - A list of allergies and intolerance to meds and other substances
    - Their history of past serious illnesses and hospitalizations, with dates included
    - A list of surgeries, with dates
    - Significant family history, especially diabetes, high blood pressure and genetic diseases
    - The name and contact information of their primary healthcare provider
- **Patients with chronic disease** should have all of the above, as well as records that include the course of their chronic disease, treatment and recent lab results.

Currently, there is an active ongoing national discussion on the importance of medical records, and most plans for healthcare reform include provisions for electronic medical records for all U.S. citizens. There are several websites that provide the electronic means to record essential medical information, including:

http://www.recordsforliving.com/HealthFrame/Ideas/Personal HealthRecord.aspx

http://www.thelivingrecord.com/ProductDetails.aspx
http://www.google.com/intl/en-US/health/tour/index.html

Healthcare planners estimate that it will be three to five years before electronic medical records will be available to everyone. In the meantime, it is essential that you have pertinent medical records available at the time of an emergency. By doing this you will greatly facilitate prompt and appropriate healthcare that avoids the problems of the missed diagnosis of a chronic disease or a severe drug allergy.

The form below has places for all the important medical information. I suggest that you complete the form below and carry a copy with you. The life you save may be your own.

MEDICAL SUMMARY

Name
Date of birth
Address
Phone

MEDICATIONS

Med	Dosage	Condition
1.		
2.		
3.		

ALLERGIES TO MEDICINES OR SUBSTANCES
1.
2.

PAST HISTORY
| Surgery | Date |
1
2.
3.

| Medical diseases | Date of onset |
1.
2.
3.

FAMILY HISTORY
1.
2.
3.

IMMUNIZATIONS
Adults, last tetanus booster:
Children, list of immunizations:

STATUS OF CHRONIC PROBLEMS
Currently being treated for:
| Illness | Doctor | Last visit |
1.
2.
3.

Blood lipids:

The course of chronic diseases can easily be summarized in a table, as below.

Date	Cholesterol	Triglycerides	HDL	LDL

Diabetes:

See *http://familydoctor.org/online/famdocen/home/common/diabetes/living/355.html* for a sample table for monitoring diabetes.

CONTACT INFORMATION

Doctor   City   Phone

1.

2.

CHAPTER TWENTY-ONE

Preparation Can Ease the Way
for You and Your Loved Ones

Anna's story

A number of years ago, a 44-year-old woman ("Anna") came to me because of recurrence of cancer of the ovary. The diagnosis of cancer had been made five years earlier. After surgery and chemotherapy, she had five good years. During that time, she was active in the American Cancer Society in its "I Can Cope" program and was accorded statewide recognition for her leadership.

I first saw Anna after she had returned to her oncologist who told her that the cancer had recurred and spread throughout her abdomen. She had a catheter placed in her abdominal cavity through which anti-cancer drugs were infused, invariably followed by severe pain. Her doctors had told her there was little hope for any cure of her condition.

Her first request to me was that the catheter be removed. In talking to Anna, it was clear that she understood that there was no other treatment for her. She had seen enough cancer patients with similar conditions that she knew that her life expectancy could be counted in a few months or even weeks. After speaking to her oncologist, I removed the catheter.

We spent an hour talking about how she could be cared for in her home. This was long before the present-day hospice service now available in most communities in the United States. I told her I would do everything possible to keep the pain in check. I also assured her I would be there if and when she needed me.

Anna was divorced and lived alone and was concerned that she not be a burden to her children. We talked about the kind of care she would get. She was clear that she didn't want to be hospitalized until the very end. I arranged for a next-door neighbor, who was a nurse, to be available to give her a shot of pain medicine every evening at bedtime. Her pain was otherwise controlled by oral medicine.

Anna continued to lose weight and became progressively weaker. The day came when she was unable to care for herself. She was barely responsive. I admitted her to the hospital and ordered that the usual admission blood tests be omitted. She was to receive only bedside nursing care. She died two days later. I was satisfied that we had faithfully followed her wishes.

Three weeks later, a very dignified older man came to my office and, with tears in his eyes, thanked me for being so kind to his daughter. This touched me deeply because I had been able to do so little medically for her. At that moment, it became clear to me that my assurance to Anna that I wouldn't abandon her— either in her physical condition or in her emotional needs—was what she needed most. I always admired Anna's courage and her approach to the end of her life. She intentionally made decisions about her care well in advance and, by doing so, retained a sense of control as we carried out her wishes.

Dying in an acute care hospital

An extensive study[15] done in England reports the challenges of dying in an acute care hospital. In England and Wales more than 68% of patients die in acute care hospitals. The authors state that the very nature of such hospitals doesn't permit optimal care to dying patients. They list a number of "challenges":

- All problems tend to become "medicalized" and are assumed to have *medical* solutions. Popular television programs tend to promote this idea.
- Unlike hospice care, the hospital is an impersonal and unfamiliar place for patients and relatives.
- It's difficult to predict how long a patient will survive, which makes it hard to know when an illness is at a terminal stage. Interestingly, doctors with the most experience generally make the most accurate predictions, whereas doctors with close relationships to their patients are less accurate in their calculations, tending to overestimate the time of survival. This may be the time for a second opinion.
- Nursing staffing changes, with legally mandated reduced working hours, have hampered the communication between doctors and patients.
- There's a lack of planning for the terminal stage of life related to the difficulty in predicting the time of death and the reluctance to say that a patient is dying. Too many dying patients remain on intravenous fluids and antibiotics and have tests that are unnecessary. Less than half the patients have a plan for palliative care. In some hospitals, 30% of patients die in intensive care units.

'It's not easy for medical caregivers, many of whom have been fighting tenaciously for a patient's life, to know the precise moment to back off intensive treatment.'

These challenges in addressing the needs of dying patients in an acute care hospital were increased by anxiety among staff in communicating with family and relatives about death. Furthermore, it's not easy for medical caregivers, many of whom have been fighting tenaciously for a patient's life, to know the precise moment to back off intensive treatment.

Pre-planning for end-of-life decisions

When I entered medical practice in 1965, essentially everything I was able to do for a patient I could handle out of my medical bag that I carried on a house call. But with the increasing technology of diagnostic tools and treatment, hospitalization became more frequently necessary. And lives were prolonged. With this development, however, came all sorts of questions about the extent of care.

Increasingly, people are facing end-of-life decisions:
- Do I want to be resuscitated if my heart stops?
- Should I place limits on medical care if I have an incurable problem?
- How do I assess quality of life as an incurable disease progresses?

As an internist, I cared for many elderly people in my practice. I tried to find the appropriate times when people were prepared to discuss their thoughts on the limits of medical care they wanted. If there were limitations, I strongly encouraged these patients to discuss the details with their family members and their pastor. This discussion included those who would make the healthcare decisions if the individual were not able. I kept a list in my office of patients who had requested limits to their care.

> *On a fall afternoon, I got a call from a nursing home that one of the persons on my list was in the emergency room after suffering a cardiac arrest. As I quickly walked the short distance from my office to the emergency room, I remembered the sweet, very bright patient and how she had made the decision to place limits on her end-of-life care. She had specifically said, "If my heart stops, don't try to restart it." Her family was aware of her decision. (Today nursing homes generally require that residents and/or family state their wishes by signing—or not signing—a "do not resuscitate" order or similar document.)*

> *On entering the cubicle in the ER, it was apparent that a full-blown cardiac resuscitation was in progress. When I told the attending medical personnel of her request, they stopped their efforts. I felt I had fulfilled my duty to her as a final act of respect and honoring her wishes.*

Medical caregivers with all good intentions are concerned that everything medically possible is being done, irrespective of the age of the patient. At these times, it's important to know the right questions and be prepared ask them. The most important questions include:
- What will be gained by this procedure or treatment?
- What if we don't do the procedure?

- Will this appreciably increase my life span?
- Is there is a good chance I will be more comfortable?
- Is it necessary to be in the hospital for this condition, or can it be treated at home?

With all the available technology, it isn't unusual for the course of treatment to take on a life of its own; one thing just seems to lead to another. There are specific times when an elderly person or family is fully entitled to ask certain questions, such as:

- When is surgery recommended?
- When is it time to move to intensive care?
- When are dialysis, feeding tubes or other procedures recommended?

The U.S. Agency for Health Research and Quality has an excellent website that lists in detail the questions that need to be asked in specific situations. The website's motto is "Questions Are the Answers" (see *http://www. ahrq.gov/questionsaretheanswer/*).

Early planning and communication with one's family are essential in preparing for issues that can arise, including the question of organ donation. A living will and power of attorney for health decisions will help. *All* of the questions cannot be answered up front. For example, if a person with terminal cancer gets pneumonia, should he or she be treated vigorously to prolong life?

Euthanasia

Such end-of-life issues inevitably raise the question of euthanasia, which is defined as an intentional overt action or omission that causes the death of another person.[16] Most states, with the exception of Oregon and Washington, have laws that prohibit anyone from aiding, abetting or encouraging suicide. These laws make it a criminal act to assist in a suicide, with the person charged with manslaughter or a felony with mandatory penalties. Several states define assisted suicide as criminal homicide.

Oregon and Washington have "Death with Dignity" laws that allow physician-assisted suicide. The law redefines assisted suicide as a medical condition that allows physicians to prescribe a lethal dose of medicine to a patient who is considered to have less than six months to live. The physician may prescribe medicine for that purpose but may not personally administer the medicine. During the first decade since the Oregon law was passed, the state has averaged 34 assisted suicides per year.

The argument for assisted suicide includes the relief from intolerable pain, permits the patient to make a choice and frees up money for the medical needs of other people. It is also a way out for patients in the terminal stages of a disease whose quality of life has become very low.

There are strong arguments against euthanasia, both theological and practical. For most people, including most physicians, assisting a patient to commit suicide is untenable. The taking of life violates the view that all human life is sacred. There is concern that assisted suicide will become a way of controlling healthcare costs. Sociologists fear that the "slippery slope" of legal euthanasia (sometimes called mercy killing) initially used only for terminal patients will evolve into ridding society of other so-called "undesirables."

In my medical practice, there were times when I understood the futility of what we could do for a person medically. With the patient and family, I literally waited with little to do until the merciful end came for a terminal patient. However, that has changed in recent years with vastly improved methods of care of the terminally ill. We now have hospice care with specialized care for patients in their last stages of life. In addition, the methods of pain control have improved markedly, including infusion pumps, which provide pain medicine through the vein under the control of the patient. Doctors now feel that there's no reason for people to suffer intolerable pain.

There are reasons why the laws in Oregon and Washington are called "Death with Dignity" laws. In surveys of older people, one of the fears they express is the loss of dignity in their last days. They visualize intensive care with tubes attached to various parts of their body and limited visitation for the family. Contrast that picture with the way my friend Willard died: at home in familiar surroundings with his loving family on hand and support services from the hospice nurses. Willard lived with dignity, and he died the same way, with his dignity preserved.

Hospice care

For the person facing terminal illness, there may come a time when further treatment will be futile. When to stop curative efforts and focus on palliative (comforting) measures is a question that needs to be faced openly, with clear and compassionate communication among the patient, family and caregivers (doctors, nurses, chaplains). When all agree that further treatment to effect a cure is futile, the goal of care shifts to providing comfort to the patient and family. This is the time when most patients are referred to hospice care.

'"How people die remains in the memories of those who live on."'

Modern hospice care was founded in England by Dame Cicely Saunders who said, "How people die remains in the memories of those who live on." Hospice care exists to make the dying process somewhat easier, addressing the physical, emotional, and spiritual needs of the dying patient and the grieving family. Hospice care is infinitely more helpful to meet these needs than if the patient is in an acute care hospital.

Much has been written about end-of-life decisions. Many professional and religious organizations list principles and guidelines. The American College of Physicians' website, *http://www.acponline.org/patients_families/end_of_life_ issues,* considers the practical issues to be faced at this time of life and enables the patient and family to better work with the professionals providing the healthcare.

A final note

Many religions view death as a transition to another (even better) life. Christians face death as a transition into a new life in the presence of God. With our families, we can make choices that ease that transition and lead to a "good death."

CHAPTER TWENTY-TWO

The Pitfalls and Possibilities of Nontraditional Medicine

How does a doctor deal with patients who want to try medical procedures and treatments that are not recognized as having a scientific basis?

Lena, 47, came to see me many years ago with lung problems. She complained of a longstanding cough, wheezing and progressive shortness of breath—the signs of emphysema or Chronic Obstructive Lung Disease (COLD). After some tests we established that she had a congenital enzyme deficiency (alpha 1 antitrypsin) that had destroyed her lungs over a period of time. At that time there was no specific treatment. We treated Lena for her symptoms but, after months passed, it was clear that she was gradually getting worse.

One day she came to the office to discuss a special treatment in Mexico. Her sister had offered to pay her train ticket to go for the treatment. She was now wondering aloud about the advisability of going and wanted my opinion.

First of all, I appreciated that she had come to talk to me to ask my advice rather than simply going off on her own. I was very aware that she was getting worse, but I had to acknowledge to her that there was nothing else I could do. Today there are both preventive protocols and treatment methods available. But this was 1974.

I asked Lena what she knew about the treatment in Mexico. She knew very little, only that her sister heard that someone else with a similar problem had gone through the treatment and was improved. Lena's breathing was clearly getting worse. There was no treatment that seemed to make it better.

Following are questions that I routinely asked myself when a medically unproven treatment was being considered:

1. Was the diagnosis certain? The diagnosis was verified by lab tests and not in doubt.
2. Had I "left no stone unturned" in seeking help for her? Consultation with a lung specialist confirmed there was no other known treatment at that time.
3. Was there any documented evidence that the unconventional treatment would help? Since we didn't know the nature of the proposed treatment, it was impossible to answer this question.
4. What was the chance that the treatment would actually harm her? This question also could not be answered, given the available data.
5. How much did the treatment cost? Was there evidence of a get-rich scheme? Again, she didn't know; furthermore, her sister was paying for it.

Ultimately, of course, Lena had to make the decision. She was well aware that I had nothing more to offer that could cure her. She clearly needed a reason to hope and, in my view, would have always second-guessed any decision not to go to Mexico. So she decided to go. I did tell her that I would be available to her when she returned.

Lena did go to Mexico. About two months later, I got a call from her husband who said she couldn't breathe, and they were going to the Emergency Room. When I met them there, I barely recognized the once familiar face of Lena. Her cheeks were rounded, and she had facial hair not seen before. I recognized these changes as typical for someone on high doses of steroids. Lena confirmed that the doctor in Mexico had placed her on steroids. She said that her breathing was better for about two weeks, then began to worsen.

Lena had a collapsed lung. Her breathing improved with re-expansion of the lung, and she was discharged home. She remained bedfast and on oxygen at home where I visited her on a regular basis until she died about six weeks later.

Lena, with the urging of her sister and in desperation to change the progressive downhill course, decided to go to Mexico where she was treated with unproven methods. The clinic in Mexico gave her high doses of steroids that temporarily improved her symptoms but within weeks led to complications that probably hastened her death.

The following story of using alternative treatment methods has a happier outcome:

Our son Ed, as a 20-year-old college student, was teaching English at a university in Chengdu, China. He and a Canadian friend played on the university basketball team. The team had unprecedented success. In the semifinal game of the season-ending tournament, Ed severely sprained his ankle. From previous experience, he knew he couldn't play the next day in the final tournament game. His Chinese coach said, "No problem, come with me." He treated the ankle with massage, acupuncture and herbal compress. To Ed's amazement, the swelling and pain quickly dissipated, and he played in the final game, helping his team to the tournament victory.

When treatment fails or an ailment goes undiagnosed, people understandably look for other sources of help for which scientific medicine has no apparent answers. In desperation, people in this circumstance seek other answers. People looking for hope in incurable conditions hear stories of medical "cures" or improvement from family and well-meaning friends. This is understandable. Hope, especially in desperate circumstances, knows no boundaries of geography or gender or even religion. Patients also may go outside usual medical treatment for a more "holistic" approach—or as a supplement to standard medical care in the hope of finding alternative ways to deal with their problem.

'Hope, especially in desperate circumstances, knows no boundaries of geography or gender or even religion.'

People in the United States are increasingly looking to complementary and alternative medicine (CAM) for medical care. In a seven-year study,[17] the number of Americans who used alternative medicine annually increased from 33.8% to 42.1% from 1990 to 1997. The therapies increasing most were herbal medicine, massage, megavitamins, self-help groups, folk remedies, energy healing and homeopathy. People most commonly sought alternative therapy for such chronic conditions as back problems, anxiety, depression and headaches. In 1997 nearly 65% of patients paid entirely out of pocket for the cost of alternative care. That same year the estimated number of visits to alternative medical practitioners was 629 million (exceeding visits to all primary care physicians) at a cost conservatively estimated at $27 billion. Practitioners of traditional medicine continue to warn that most of these approaches to treatment lack scientific proof by high-quality clinical studies.

Modern medicine is based on clearly defined scientific methods that prove its effectiveness. When first introduced, however, many modern medicines and treatments lacked scientific proof of their value. The best of medical care fails in some cases, either because there are no known answers or because of errors. When the diagnosis is obscure or the treatment ineffective, people turn to alternative and unproven modes of treatment. CAM is gradually finding more acceptance.

'Quacks'

Organized medicine has rightly attempted to protect the unsuspecting public from unscrupulous "quacks" who tend to take advantage of people's fears and ignorance. Opportunities for quacks abound in situations where standard medicine has no ready answers and where suggested treatment is confusing or controversial. Non-medical persons also may be perplexed about what constitutes adequate qualifications for medical practitioners.

Some quacks have gained considerable notoriety. Here's a famous example from a century ago:

> In 1917 "Dr." John Brinkley, a former snake-oil sales-
> man, bought a medical diploma from Eclectic Med-
> ical University of Kansas City.[18] While working in an
> abattoir, he noticed the vigorous mating of goats
> before slaughter. When a farmer named Stittsworth
> came to see him complaining of loss of sexual
> prowess, Brinkley jokingly suggested that he needed
> a goat testicle transplant. The farmer replied, "So
> Doc, put 'em in." Brinkley crushed a bit of goat testi-
> cle and injected it into Stittsworth's testicle.
> Sitttsworth returned several weeks later loudly pro-
> claiming his improved ability to perform sexually.
> When his wife had a son, he named him "Billy" in
> honor of the goat.
>
> The news of the procedure spread quickly, and Brinkley
> became a busy man. In a decade, he did more than
> 16,000 procedures at $750 each, becoming immensely
> wealthy. Brinkley effectively stifled dissent by stating
> that the treatment was very effective in intelligent men
> but worked poorly in stupid men. Brinkley's license to
> practice medicine was taken away after Dr. Fishbein of
> the American Medical Association denounced him as a
> charlatan. As a means of regaining his license, Brinkley
> ran for governor of Kansas, promising free medical
> clinics for all. He lost in a close election. On his
> deathbed, he reportedly said, "If Fishbein goes to
> heaven, I don't want to go there."[19]

A quack is any person who fraudulently practices medicine, claiming knowledge or skill he/she does not possess (*New World Dictionary, Second College Edition*).

Quacks have been the bane of the medical profession since the time of Hippocrates. Quacks use various tactics in an effort to attract clients. The following list identifies 11 traits:

1. Uses scare tactics.
2. Views the medical establishment as a conspiracy preventing the use of the methods or remedies they espouse.
3. Rejects standard care.
4. Is secretive about cures and proofs of effectiveness.
5. Stands to profit from promotion and sales of products or services.
6. Uses unrecognized credentials and is unlicensed and unregulated.
7. Tends to distort and simplify.
8. Uses pseudomedical jargon: "detoxify, purify, revitalize."
9. Offers simple tests to "prove" you need the treatment.
10. Wears the cloak of science: "Studies are under way," "Science doesn't have all the answers," etc.
11. When treatment fails, often says: "If only you had come sooner."

Traditional medicine is fallible

Traditional medicine, it must be noted, is far from infallible. In one of the most tragic examples, more than 10,000 people worldwide have severe birth defects because their mothers were prescribed thalidomide for nausea during their pregnancies in the 1950s; it was later learned that the thalidomide caused birth deformities. These persons are easily recognizable today because of a characteristic defect: severely stunted upper limbs, with some individuals having only "flippers" instead of arms. The tragedy of thalidomide also touched the medical profession. An obstetrician acquaintance of mine had to leave obstetrics because he had prescribed thalidomide for a number of patients.

'Traditional medicine, it must be noted, is far from infallible.'

Therapies and modes of treatment find favor, then sometimes fall into disrepute. Critics of CAM tend to overlook the shortcomings and failures of Western medicine. We may too easily succumb to the human tendency to compare the ideal of the method we favor to the worst reports of the method we don't favor. But, as a *Lancet* editorial suggests, "Before doctors rush to condemn the weak evidence underpinning these therapies, they should pause and consider the record of orthodox medicine."[20]

The U.S. Institute of Medicine estimates that there are 94,000 "preventable" deaths per year in hospitals. The table below shows the relative risk of dying from a "preventable death" in a hospital compared with other everyday occurrences.

Safety Hazards and Everyday Possibilities
(Chances per 1 million opportunities)

AIDS infection from a blood transfusion	0.07
All "heads" on 20 consecutive coin tosses	1
Death of a commercial airline passenger	2.4
Death from general anesthesia	7.5
Death from a motor vehicle accident	187
Preventable hospital deaths	208

The Agency for Healthcare Research and Quality
http://webmm.ahrq.gov/dykarchivecase.aspx?dykID=1
Accessed April 16, 2005

This table shows that for every million passengers on a commercial airline, 2.4 will die and for every million patients in a hospital, 208 will die from deaths that could have been prevented. The chance of dying a preventable death as a patient in a hospital is *86* times greater than from dying as a passenger on a commercial flight.

The process from alternative medicine to full acceptance

Folklore and "old wives' tales" about how to cure illness have existed throughout human history. For most of those millennia the ways of caring for sick people evolved through serendipity and trial and error. Modern science and scientific medicine are relatively recent arrivals on the human stage. By contemporary definitions, virtually all medical care before 1700 was "alternative"—without scientific proof of efficacy. The process from folklore to acceptance in modern medicine is long and arduous as the following account of digitalis illustrates.

Digitalis

For centuries, doctors described a medical condition of fluid accumulation throughout the bodies of patients that

> puffed their bodies into grotesque shapes, squeezed their lungs, and finally brought slow but inexorable death. As the disease progressed, a watery liquid filtered into every available space and expanded it like a balloon. Sometimes the liquid—quarts and gallons of it—made arms and legs swell so that they were immovable. Sometimes it poured into the abdomen to form a tremendous paunch. Sometimes it waterlogged the lung cavity and thereby made it impossible for the victim to breathe unless he sat bolt upright all day and all night.[21]

This condition, formerly known as hydrops or dropsy, is now called congestive heart failure. For centuries, healers sought treatment for this condition of a failing heart. Tea made from the dried leaf of the garden herb foxglove, *digitalis purura alba,* was noted to slow and strengthen the heartbeat and help rid the body of excess fluid. Dr. Withering,[22] one of the early pioneers in its use, was criticized when he first began using digitalis. Fellow physicians considered this treatment without basis in the science of medicine of the day. Digitalis, however, gradually became accepted for use in treating congestive heart failure.

When I began medical practice in 1965, digitalis was available only as digitalis *folia,* the pulverized leaf of the plant compressed into tablets. The administration of this form of digitalis was tricky, with a small margin between a therapeutic level and toxicity (with nausea, vomiting and heart rhythm problems). Later researchers identified and synthesized the active ingredient in digitalis. These synthesized forms of digitalis became available commercially, making possible the accurate adjustment of doses in specific patients. The road from alternative medicine to full acceptance spanned a couple of centuries.

Digitalis represents a common sequence for acceptance of a new medicine or treatment that includes: (1) the discovery of a naturally occurring substance with beneficial medical properties; (2) scientific testing to prove its efficacy; (3) identification of the severity and incidence of side effects; (4) identification of the active ingredient; (5) synthesis of the active ingredient; and (6) final field testing, leading to approval by the U.S. Food & Drug Administration. Only then is the medicine or treatment ready for marketing. This process usually takes years. With digitalis, it took about 200 years from its first discovery to the synthesis of the active ingredient.

Conclusion

Western practitioners *assume* that traditional, science-based healthcare is superior to complementary and alternative disciplines. Traditional medicine, in its attempt to control the quality of medical care, insists on scientific evidence regarding the efficacy and safety of treatment procedures and medicines. Without this evidence, any treatment is suspect. Organized traditional medicine rightly seeks to protect a medically unsophisticated public against quacks and charlatans.

However, an arm's-length, dispassionate look at the results of traditional medicine should give us pause. In our assumption of superiority, we tend to compare the ideal of traditional medicine to the stories of failure in other forms of practice. All of us in the traditional medical field, as well as strong adherents outside it, need to be humbled by the incidence of in-hospital deaths, drug reactions and failed treatments. Too often, we have no answers for patients with chronic and incurable diseases.

Patients and families increasingly seek out practitioners of alternative medicine—both as part of their routine care and as part of their quest for answers to problems for which there are no ready solutions in orthodox medicine.

As suggested above, many modern medicines started as scientifically unproven alternative treatments. The process from alternative to scientifically proven tends to be long indeed. Traditional medicine has controlled the purse strings of scientific research and has allowed few funds for the necessary studies that would prove or disprove the effectiveness of CAM. In so doing, people are making choices about using or not using CAM without sufficient knowledge. Historically, as noted, yesterday's alternative medicine may become tomorrow's orthodox treatment. By limiting research into selected areas of CAM, we may miss that next breakthrough that will ease pain and suffering and extend useful life. Encouragingly in recent years, research money is becoming more available for these purposes.

CHAPTER TWENTY-THREE

Why Does Healthcare Cost So Much?

What are we getting for our money?

People in the United States spend, on average, about 50% more for healthcare than other developed countries.

Cost of healthcare per person per year in U.S. dollars:

- Australia $2,903
- Canada $3,003
- Germany $2,996
- New Zealand $1,886
- United Kingdom $2,331
- **United States**   **$5,635**

The Commonwealth Fund Report, April 2006

What do we get for the extra money? Many Americans are certain that we have the best healthcare in the world. But the numbers don't bear that out when measured by the usual parameters of healthcare. In comparison with other developed countries, the United States is:

- **Forty-second in life expectancy.** Even though life expectancy in the United States has been gradually increasing in recent years, this country is falling further behind in comparison with other developed countries. Japan has the highest life expectancy at 81.4, with the U.S.

at 78. Zimbabwe has the lowest life expectancy at 39.5 years. Researchers cite the factors that lower the U.S. life expectancy including the number of people who have inadequate healthcare because they're uninsured, increasing obesity and racial differences.[23]

- **Thirty-seventh in infant mortality rate (IMR),** defined as the number of deaths per thousand infants under 1 year of age. The IMR in the U.S. is 6.4 compared with 2.8 in Sweden, Iceland and Japan. The highest reported IMR in 2007 was Angola where 184 babies out of 1,000 births died under 1 year of age. I polled eight mothers in a village clinic in Cambodia. They reported that 17 of their 33 live babies died before their fifth birthday during and after the Pol Pot holocaust.

- **Twenty-fourth in healthy life years.** Healthy aging requires protection from exposure to unhealthy conditions and diseases, information to help people prevent disease, early diagnosis and proper treatment. As populations age, an increasing proportion will become disabled. The ability to properly care for persons with chronic illness and postpone the onset of disability is a measure of the adequacy of the healthcare system.

High administrative costs

One of the reasons for the added expenditures is that in this country we spend 21% of the total cost of healthcare for administration. In contrast, the cost of administration in the government Medicare/Medicaid program is 4.7%. This difference of 16.3% amounts to about to about $350 billion— enough to provide healthcare to everyone in the nation. This administrative cost goes to people who sell insurance, to those who work on new insurance products, and to profit for the insurance company. Paul Krugman, *New York Times* editorial economist, estimates there are 2 million people whose job it is to either get the money for medical services provided or who work for insurance companies to determine the eligibility of the claims.

Cost to practitioners

What does the cost of administration mean to doctors? U.S. physicians spend about one-eighth of their time on administration (1999 figures) with an average cost of $269 per capita. The comparable numbers for Canadian doctors is about one-twelfth of their time spent and $55 per capita.[24]

In 1999, of the 11.7 million people working in the U.S. healthcare industry, 27.3% worked in administrative and clerical services. This was an increase from 18.2% thirty years earlier. In Canada the increase in the percentage of administrative healthcare workers has been appreciably less; from 1971 to 1996 the percentage of people working in administrative and clerical services increased from 16% to 19.1%. These numbers do not include insurance employees.

'Administrative and clerical time
is increased in the U.S. with its system
of multiple insurers as opposed to
a single-payer system.'

Administrative and clerical time is increased in the U.S. with its system of multiple insurers as opposed to a single-payer system. The many insurance companies with diverse plans require a great deal of time and many personnel to sort out the eligibility, differing co-payments, referral networks and methods of approval.

Hospital costs

Dr. Uwe E. Reinhardt, professor of economics at Princeton, writing in the *NYTimes* blog, *Economix,* has a concise and excellent discussion of hospital reimbursement for medical services.[25] There are three different methods of reimbursement for hospital services: Medicare/Medicaid, private insurance and uninsured.

Medicare reimbursement to hospitals is based on DRGs (diagnosis-related groups). This method of payment assumes that the cost of a hospitalization will be relative to the disease or condition being treated. Congress then sets the schedule of reimbursement, according to DRGs. Hospital lobbyists try to get the rates set at the average cost per diagnosis.

Patients without insurance are charged the full non-discounted rates for the hospital services. Hospitals negotiate with uninsured patients on an individual basis (for example, the Amish; see Chapter 24). Private insurers negotiate with hospitals for a per diem rate per diagnosis that is usually set slightly higher than the hospital cost. Thus private insurers cover some of the cost not reimbursed by Medicare and the uninsured.

Each hospital has a master list where they list their charges per diagnosis that is specific to that hospital. The cost for procedures may vary as much as tenfold for a given procedure. For instance, in California hospitals the cost for an appendectomy to the insurer varied from $1,800 to $13,700. Professor Reinhardt calls the method of reimbursement for medical services to hospitals "chaos behind a veil of secrecy." All this is reminiscent of Churchill's description in 1939 of the Soviet Union—"a riddle wrapped in a mystery inside an enigma."

The 'cost' of chronic illness

Most chronic diseases—unlike an injury, appendicitis or pneumonia—make their appearance slowly and insidiously. Diabetes is a prime example of a chronic disease with a slow onset. The Centers for Disease Control estimated in 2007 that there were 23.6 million diabetics in this country, with nearly one-third of these undiagnosed. In addition, they estimate there are 57 million persons with pre-diabetes who will develop the disease if they don't change their lifestyle.

The cost of diabetes in 2007 was estimated to be $116 billion in direct medical costs. In addition, the estimated cost of loss of productivity due to absenteeism, early disability and death was $58 billion. Medical costs average 2.3 times higher for diabetics than non-diabetics.

It is essential that individuals with diabetes have a basic understanding of the disease and know how to monitor and control it. With proper control, the complications can be prevented or their onset delayed, hospitalizations prevented and productive life prolonged. Persons with diabetes and other chronic diseases will need to change their mindset and adjust to the idea that they have a medical problem that will not go away and needs long-term care.

High blood pressure (HBP) is another chronic problem, affecting an estimated 72 million Americans. The complications of HBP can be catastrophic, with a 50% greater likelihood of a stroke or heart attack. Blood pressure can be controlled in virtually all cases. Only 39%, however, are adequately controlled. Most patients with HBP have no symptoms, pointing to the need for routine blood-pressure screening.

The annual average cost of healthcare for an employee with uncontrolled HBP is 2½ times higher than for those with controlled blood pressure ($619 to $217 per patient per month). Nationally, the annual cost of HBP is estimated at more than $66 billion.

The epidemic of obesity in the United States is the major contributing factor in the high incidence of HBP and diabetes. Obesity is increasing at alarming rates, including in young children, which will place further stress on the U.S. healthcare system. Most of us know all this, and we know the means to controlling weight, but we procrastinate. See Chapter 25 on wellness and taking charge of one's own health.

Unnecessary medical care

Shannon Brownlee,[26] author of *Overtreated: Why Too Much Medicine Is Making Us Sicker and Poorer* (Bloomsbury, 2007), says the major reason the cost of healthcare is so high is that most Americans get too much care. Tests and imaging are done because they are available. As in the story cited in the chapter on defensive medicine, patients often insist on multiple tests where simple and inexpensive testing would suffice without the loss of quality.

Imaging scans are the fastest-growing segment of healthcare. The American College of Radiology (ACR) notes the "skyrocketing" cost of scanning, with the costs of CT (computerized tomography), MRI (magnetic resonance imaging) and PET (positron emission tomography) scans increasing at double the rate of other healthcare costs. The ACR, through its MEDIC (medical excellence in diagnostic imaging campaign) program,[27] is pushing to establish quality standards. It quotes evidence that physicians who have financial interest in the scans (CT, MRI, PET) order twice as many scans as physicians without any financial interest. Further, according to ACR, many non-radiology scans don't meet safety standards, and the incidence of misinterpretation is higher among non-radiologists.

Rapid developments in the technology of scans have fueled this expansion. Patients are aware of the availability of the scans; many want the latest available.

Most of us think of brain scans as looking for tumors or other pathologies, such as cysts or cancer. Recent advances in brain scans now claim the ability to explore non-anatomical functions, such as feelings, anger, memory and motivation. This raises a whole new area of exploration that has ethical and healthcare cost implications.[28]

Very few scans are 100% accurate. In the course of diagnostic testing, there is usually little mention of the possibility of a false positive test (a scan that show abnormalities when there is no disease or condition present) or false negative test (a scan that shows no abnormality, even though the disease or condition is clearly present). Because of the possibility of false positives, further testing to confirm the original test is usually done. In surveying the literature, it is difficult to find studies that give firm answers to the incidence of false positive and false negative tests.

If a doctor suggests a scan, the patient needs to ask several questions:
- Is there risk in doing the test?
- What are we looking for?

Tell the doctor that you understand there are false positive and false negative tests and ask:

- What do we do if the scan is positive?
- What do we do if the scan is negative?
- How much does the scan cost?

We've talked about scans. There are other areas where we may be overtreated. We're subjected to intense advertising about the use of drugs and how life and health can be improved if only we take a new medicine. In many ways we've come to feel that there must be a *medical* cure for whatever ails us. We take medicine for backache and heartburn; for high blood pressure, high cholesterol and high blood sugar; and for erectile dysfunction and benign prostatic hypertrophy.

'We're subjected to intense advertising about the use of drugs and how life and health can be improved if only we take a new medicine.'

In a recent study[29] of the incidence of lower back pain, the authors noted that the reported incidence of lower back pain was 10% less in East Germany than in West Germany. Ten years after reunification, however, the incidence was essentially the same. The authors speculate that "much of the increase in prevalence rates [in East Germany] was due to dissemination of back-related attitudes and beliefs from the more 'medicalized' West Germany."

The law of supply and demand doesn't work

Is healthcare a right of every citizen or a privilege for those who have the money to buy care? All (yes, all) other developed countries in the world take the former position and provide healthcare as a right of all citizens.

In 2003 my wife, Marilyn, and I went to work for nine months as volunteers in a peace center in England. The day we arrived we registered at the local general practitioner's office. The following morning Marilyn awoke with swelling and pain over the right side of her face, as well as her scalp. She went to see the GP who diagnosed shingles; because of the possibility of eye involvement she sent Marilyn to the downtown eye clinic. Within three hours she saw two doctors and received four prescriptions, all at no cost. At no time did anyone involved in Marilyn's care ask about insurance or who would pay the bill. Because of the prompt and appropriate treatment, Marilyn rapidly recovered from a potentially debilitating problem.

Two years later Irish friends were spending three months in study in the United States. On the first day of school their 8-year-old daughter fell off some monkey bars and broke her arm. Her father later emotionally told me that, before the ER personnel agreed to see his daughter, they insisted on knowing who would pay. He had become accustomed to the idea that healthcare was a right of citizenship and was dismayed at the U.S. ordeal of getting medical attention.

In the United States we have tended to view healthcare as a commodity to buy and sell, with profits made for the providers of healthcare. Healthcare, if viewed as a commodity, should be subject to the law of supply and demand.

Is healthcare a commodity that is to be bought and sold and a profit made? The fear in this country is that if healthcare is made available to all at affordable prices (taking healthcare off the commodity market), there will be overutilization of services. This is contrary to the experience of other countries. Americans pay 2–3 times more per person for healthcare, yet the measures of health in the U.S. are lower than in most other developed countries.

> *In 2008 Marilyn and I spent a lovely three days in Stratford, Ontario, at the Shakespeare festival. While there I asked a number of local people about their healthcare. Two people mentioned long waits for elective surgery, such as joint replacement and arthritic complaints. There was general satisfaction otherwise, and people looked at me in disbelief if not incredulity when I asked if they would trade for the U.S. system. I asked about MRIs. The small city of Stratford doesn't have an MRI. Residents drive either to Waterloo or London, Ontario, and their appointment may be at 12:15 a.m. because the machine is operated 24 hours a day.*

Contrast the experience in Ontario with the typical situation in the U.S. Here the decision of whether to buy an MRI machine at a cost of about 1 million dollars is a business decision. The key question is if the machine can be paid for. Will there be enough procedures to make the payments? Thus there is subtle pressure on physicians (or not so subtle if the physician profits from the MRI procedures) to order enough procedures to have the convenience of an MRI in the community. The decision to order an MRI usually takes little thought on the part of the physician or the insured patient. On the other hand, if the patient needs to travel 50 or more miles for the procedure, the decision will likely be made with more thought to justify it. Studies verify that the number of MRI procedures (and other modalities of testing) per capita is relative to the prevalence of MRI machines in an area.

How about the number of doctors in a community? Won't the cost of healthcare come down if there are more doctors? If the law of supply and demand works, this should be the case. David Goodman,[30] an investigator for the *Dartmouth Atlas of Health Care 1999,* cites studies that indicate that an increased density of doctors in a community does not improve the quality of healthcare. However, there is clear evidence that what it does is *increase the cost* of healthcare.

The study compared the cities of Miami and Minneapolis. Miami had 40% more doctors per capita and 50% more specialists than Minneapolis. The Medicare patients in Miami had more hospitalizations, more expensive procedures and more specialist consultations—and they were more likely to spend time in the intensive care unit in the last six months of life than Minneapolis patients. Yet the elderly in Miami do not live longer than Minneapolis residents. Despite the greater number of doctors in Miami—with, presumably, greater availability to their patients—patient satisfaction with their medical care was about equal.

Defensive medicine

Defensive medicine, as covered in more depth in Chapter 2, is the deviation from sound medical practice on the part of doctors in order to decrease the probability of a lawsuit for malpractice. The cost of defensive medicine is estimated as high as 3% of the total cost of healthcare. Three percent may not sound like much, but it amounts to $60 billion of the annual bill for medical services in the U.S.

'Defensive medicine contributes in several ways to added costs.'

Defensive medicine contributes in several ways to added costs. First, the doctor, in order to head off a lawsuit, orders additional treatment or tests that have virtually no value in diagnosis or treatment. As there is no recognized standard of care for many problems, physicians, in practicing defensive medicine, too often make decisions based on what a plaintiff's attorney *might* ask in a courtroom. In the absence of a uniform standard of care, the adequacy of care is decided by a jury of non-medical persons. Doctors understandably remain uneasy with this system.

Second, doctors will be quick to point out the high cost of malpractice insurance. *Medical Economics,* the business journal for doctors, has a regular feature article on malpractice, attesting to its importance. Malpractice premiums are relative to the risk of the specialty, the location of the practitioner and any previous lawsuit. Several years ago malpractice premiums hit an all-time high for most doctors, with decreases in some areas since then. In 2004 the highest cost of malpractice insurance was in Miami, Florida, with annual premiums of $65,000 for internists and $227,000 for general surgeons. Costs are somewhat less in other cities. These premium costs must be paid so the doctor can stay in business. Most hospitals require any attending doctor to carry malpractice insurance.[31]

Third, physicians may try to avoid malpractice suits by quickly referring a patient to a specialist, purely to protect himself or herself. One doctor said that some patients walking through the door immediately appear to be a "malpractice suit waiting to happen." This is particularly true with a patient with a previous history of malpractice litigation. The natural inclination is to almost automatically refer that patient to a specialist—at added expense.

Lifestyle issues

It is generally accepted (and confirmed by other doctors and healthcare providers) that 70% of the costs of healthcare in this country are due to the lifestyle choices people make. Leading this list is smoking, alcoholism, obesity, lack of exercise and improper diet. Seventy percent! Clearly, this factor alone can lower the cost of healthcare (and improve the quality of life) more significantly than all other factors combined. Again, see Chapter 25 on wellness. There is immense potential for feeling better *and* reducing the cost of healthcare through the choices we make.

Duplication of efforts

Most patients at some time or another have had experience with lost or unavailable laboratory test results. Too frequently the practice is simply to repeat the test. See Chapters 3 and 20 on medical records; they stress the importance of carrying copies of key medical records with you.

The dwindling availability of PCPs

The American College of Physicians expressed concern about the decreasing numbers of young doctors entering primary medicine. The availability of primary care physicians is essential to maintain the quality of healthcare and control its cost. See Chapter 18 on PCPs.

Conclusion

The U.S. system of healthcare in reality is no system at all but rather a hodge-podge of fragmented care where too many decisions about the purchase of expensive equipment and the high rate of utilization of expensive tests become business decisions instead of decisions based on medical necessity.

In my opinion, in years past, higher values were placed on honor and service. These basic motivating factors were followed by providers of health services, whether individual or institutional. If there was a failure to provide the best services, it was a source of consternation, even shame, and there was impetus to fix what had gone wrong.

All too often, these values have been replaced by the need to turn a profit. This may be particularly true of provider institutions or huge corporations, including pharmaceutical houses and insurance companies

Healthcare in this country is being priced out of reach for millions of Americans. It will take the best organizational minds and determined political will to find the best combination of private and public organizational mix to provide decent, affordable healthcare to all. The planners will need to give careful attention to more efficient delivery of healthcare, the establishment of experience-based standards of care, easily available medical records and a new commitment to effective preventive medicine.

It is the thesis of this book that no matter what national healthcare plan evolves, costs will need to be controlled. Part of that cost containment will come as informed consumers of their own healthcare become much more involved in their healthcare decisions. This will be a win/win situation that not only decreases costs but also improves the quality of care.

CHAPTER TWENTY-FOUR

No Health Insurance:
How the Amish Do It

Introduction

In 2004, I moved to a community in northern Indiana where many Amish live.[32] I have become accustomed to seeing black Amish buggies in and around my community and hearing the mesmerizing sound of a clip-clopping horse go by. When most of us think of the Amish, we visualize people with quaint, old-fashioned bonnets and broad-brimmed hats; colorful quilts; and one-day barn raisings.

An estimated 230,000 Amish live in the United States. Most of them don't buy insurance, including health insurance, choosing to trust in a loving and benevolent God—and God's people—to care for them.

Most Amish also continue to practice strict separation from "the world" and modernity. They don't buy cars or tractors— and refuse to be connected to the electrical grid or have landline telephones because it would connect them too closely to the non-Amish world. Cell phones are generally permissible *if* deemed necessary to conduct business.

The Amish are connected to each other through strong family and community ties. Bishop districts are the basic unit, typically with a single congregation of about 40 families.

When the district grows larger, the Amish spawn another district. There are about 160 bishop districts in northern Indiana. The geographical size of the district depends on the concentration of Amish families. A district may be several square miles in size or as small as a half-mile stretch along a country road. Amish ministers and bishops—always men—are chosen through a process of voting for candidates, whereupon they are chosen by "lot."[33]

> *The Amish value and find meaning in their work. Two Chinese medical professors were visiting our Ohio home a number of years ago. They had heard of the Amish, and I offered to take them to meet my friend Jonas. They readily accepted. When we arrived at Jonas' house he was just ready to take an electric fencer to a pasture, so the Chinese professors climbed into his buggy with him and rode the two miles with me following in the car.*
>
> *I don't know what they talked about in the buggy ride, but when I caught up with them, Jonas asked, "What do the Chinese people think about the Amish?" One of the professors replied, "We think the Amish are hardworking and honest." I looked on as Jonas, a humble Amish farmer, struggled to contain his pride.*

Overall in the United States, more that 60% of personal bankruptcies are related to medical bills, more than half of which involve people who *have* health insurance. Just not enough. So how do the Amish do it without *any* insurance? Bankruptcies among the Amish are virtually unheard of—related to healthcare bills or for any other reason.[34] In view of the high cost of healthcare, I was curious how the Amish cope. So I did some research—and some visiting.

'Bankruptcies among the Amish are virtually unheard of— related to healthcare bills or for any other reason.'

I talked to two Amish bishops and an Amish naturopath. They all shared freely regarding their experience with healthcare. They deflected any attention from themselves personally and tended to downplay praise of the Amish way of life. All of them preferred not to be identified by their real name because that would set them apart from their community.

In addition, I talked to two "English" people who work almost daily with the Amish and their healthcare needs— Kate Shantz, a nurse/midwife, and Cindy Siedler, director of Immergrun, an organization that negotiates for discount healthcare services on behalf of the Amish.

Amish attitudes toward healthcare

The way Amish view health and healthcare starts with their basic beliefs. The practical expression of their faith was placed on full view to the world after the West Nickel Mines School tragedy in the fall of 2006 when a distraught English neighbor man killed five young Amish school girls and seriously injured five more.[35] Even in times of tragedy, the Amish believe that God is in control. They recognize the presence of evil in the world due to bad human choices. They believe that good can come out of evil and tragedy and saw evidence of that as the outside world noted their forgiveness of the perpetrator of the crime at West Nickel Mines School. Many Amish say the Lord's Prayer several times a day; after the tragedy, some found comfort in repeating the phrase from that prayer, "Thy will be done" many times a day.

With the belief that a kind and caring God is in control, the Amish place their trust in the providence of God. Accordingly, they don't buy any kind of insurance. In times of need they have always looked to the community for help. They traditionally care for their orphans and old people without relying on the government or outside social services. In recognition of their self-sufficiency in covering the cost to their own needy, the Amish are not required to pay into the U.S. Social Security system. They rely on each other within the community. The most obvious visual picture of this mutual aid is the gathering of dozens of men[36] and women for a barn raising after an Amish family's barn has burned down. The men work on the new barn, while the women prepare a bountiful meal. Children also help.

The Amish see good health as a gift from God and search for meaning in what happens to them. An Amish man told me that he prayed daily to understand the meaning of his extended illness, believing that something good would come of it. They continue to look to home remedies rather than running to the doctor for every ache or sniffle. The bishop's wife told me how she treated her 4-year-old child with a "bad cold" with mustard plasters over a period of three days before he improved. Bishop T couldn't remember the last time he had seen a doctor and didn't know the name of his doctor.

In accordance with their reliance on the providence of God, the Amish have little interest in such preventive healthcare measures as immunizations, Pap smears or breast exams. Too, their large families attest to their avoidance of any form of birth control.

The Amish have practiced a way of laying on of hands for healing. *Brauche,* also called powwowing, is practiced by persons believed to be especially gifted by God for this purpose.[37] Bishop H says his mother was one of these persons. She wanted to train him in this tradition, but he wasn't interested. *Brauche* involves gentle massage that locates the problem and relieves the pain. Some practitioners use charms or magical words at the bedside. Treatment by *brauchers* is free, but donations are accepted.

Bishop H says that the practice of traditional healing using *brauche* has been used less in the last number of years. People now tend to go more to doctors and other healers, such as chiropractors, naturopaths and herbalists. Bishop H said there's a man in his church who has the gift. This *braucher* can take on the pain of others. If he sits beside someone in church who has a stomach ache, *he* gets the stomach ache and the ill person feels better. For a fussy baby, 30 seconds of quiet massage will often quiet the infant.

> *At 8 years of age, I was playing at my grandfather's house and sprained my ankle. My grandmother urged my Amish Mennonite grandfather to heal the ankle with "powwowing." I recall clearly that he said some unintelligible words as he gently massaged the ankle. I soon went back to playing without pain. My parents were not happy with the powwowing, and it soon fell out of favor in our community because it was suspected to be "of the Devil" and related to witchcraft.*

The Amish are careful about how they spend their money; most live a simple and frugal lifestyle. Amish take note of what in their view appears as opulence in hospitals. Amishman S.S. Stoltzfus in an editorial in a Pennsylvania newspaper read by many Amish took note that the cost of healthcare for Amish had doubled in the prior four years. As the causes of the escalating costs, he cited building programs that include large parking garages, impressive offices and entrance lobbies, high executive salaries, and huge hospital profits.[38]

'The Amish generally refuse to buy an item until they have the money to pay for it.'

The Amish generally refuse to buy an item until they have the money to pay for it. There's an old (possibly apocryphal) story about an Amish man and his wife who were buying a farm. When it came time to pay for the farm, the man asked his wife to fetch the crock full of money. But when the money was counted there was only $27,000 instead of the agreed-upon price of $30,000. The Amish man turned to his wife and said, "Ach, you brought the wrong crock."

Mutual aid

Mutual aid is a vital practice in the Amish community just as it was among their 16th-century Anabaptist ancestors. Hans Leopold, a Swiss Anabaptist martyr of 1528, said of the brethren, "If they know of any one who is in need, whether or not he is a member of their church, they believe it is their duty out of love to God to render help and aid."[39] (The Swiss Brethren and the Amish in Europe divided in 1693, largely over the issue of "shunning." Jakob Ammann took a literal view of biblical passages on that point, while the other Anabaptist groups took a more symbolic and moderate view. From that point forward the group that endorsed shunning as a church discipline became known as the Amish.)[40]

In many Amish congregations, when a major hospital expense came up, a deacon negotiated with the hospital to get a discounted price with the promise to pay cash at the time of discharge from the hospital. The Amish were aware that Medicare and insurance companies received generous discounts on their hospital bills not available to people who are self-insured or those without insurance, and they tried to get the same discount. They found a great deal of variation among the various hospitals and healthcare providers in the community with regard to discounts and charges for the same services.

The Amish naturally began to go to specific healthcare providers with the best prices. For example, a hospital outside the immediate community was known to have a much lower price for hip replacement. Lists were drawn up that helped people decide where their healthcare would be less expensive.

The practice of helping each other in times of need extends to paying medical bills similar to a barn burning down. The deacon would make the financial need known to the congregation, and members would voluntarily contribute. If the medical bill is small, the family takes care of it. For larger bills, the local congregations get involved and help pay the bill by freewill offerings. As noted above, there are 160 Amish congregations in Elkhart and LaGrange, Indiana, counties that are subdivided into six groups. If the bill is large, the need is presented in neighboring clusters of congregations. In the case of huge bills, Amish in Indiana ask for help from Amish congregations in Ohio and Pennsylvania. I asked the bishop how people respond in such cases. He replied, "They give generously because they feel they may be next to need similar help."

'In the case of huge bills, Amish in Indiana ask for help from Amish congregations in Ohio and Pennsylvania.'

In some Amish communities there is a practice of benefit ice cream socials or fund-raising sales. Recently an Amish housewife was kicked in the face by a horse, causing severe injuries and near blindness. At last word the community was planning a benefit auction where people would donate household and other goods, with the proceeds going to help the family.

The aforementioned bishop, H, has seen the way the Amish pay for their healthcare change dramatically in the last several years. The major difference has been the ability to more effectively negotiate with hospitals and doctors about the charges. Earlier the local hospital agreed to a 20% discount, which seemed like a breakthrough until the Amish discovered that the charges *started* higher. So they decided it wasn't a great deal after all. As a community they began to go to other area hospitals asking for the same discount that Medicare gives—about 30%. Several years ago the community joined together with other Amish communities, which provides them with some leverage to get discounts from healthcare providers. Bishop H told me I needed to talk to Cindy at Immergrun.

Immergrun

A week later I went to talk to Cindy Siedler at Immergrun. The office is in a single-story, strip mall-like building containing several office suites near Toledo, Ohio. All the doors to the offices open directly to the outside without an inside hallway.

In 1983 surgeon Edwin Nirdlinger started an outpatient clinic for self-pay people without health insurance for uncomplicated hernia repair. This appealed particularly to working folks because of the policy of same-day surgery, no hospitalization and return to work in seven days. The $1,000 charge was a fraction of the usual charge in a hospital of $4,000 to $5,000.

The staff of the clinic was astounded by the number of Amish patients who soon began showing up for surgery. The Amish and other "plain" people came by the vanloads from the Amish communities in Ohio and Indiana. It was about a three-hour drive for both. Soon the staff made arrangements for nearby motel rooms to accommodate the large numbers of out-of-town patients.

Initially, Dr. Nirdlinger was the only surgeon. Later other surgeons joined the group. Local hospitals in the Toledo area agreed to give discounted rates to Amish patients. Hospital officials consented to this arrangement because they want to fill their beds—and because the Amish pay on discharge without the hassle of insurance forms.

In 2002 Dr. Nirdlinger started a non-profit organization (Immergrun) with the stated goals to: "Negotiate quality health care at affordable prices for Anabaptists who don't have health insurance (out of religious conviction) and to promote wellness."

Because of the clientele, he practiced less defensive medicine. For example, if a patient came in with typical symptoms of carpal tunnel syndrome, he did not routinely do the nerve conduction studies (EMG) usually done before surgery to verify the diagnosis. The omission of EMG saved $1,500 to $2,000.

Immergrun (German for *evergreen*) now has more than 50,000 subscribers from Ohio, Indiana and Illinois. Hospital officials and other healthcare providers pay attention when Ms. Siedler, representing Immergrun, comes to discuss discounted rates. Ms. Siedler, negotiating with a hospital finance officer for potentially hundreds of Amish, has much more leverage than a deacon representing individual cases. Immergrun currently had discount agreements with 40 hospitals and more than 200 healthcare providers.

The individual who registers with Immergrun must be a member of an Amish congregation or the child of someone who is. Immergrun charges 7% in administrative fees to pay for office and travel expenses and the salaries of two and a half employees.[41] An Amish family who signs up with Immergrun pays no subscription fee. Participants pay their share of the administrative cost only when they use the service.[42]

In 2008 Immergrun paid charges of more than $3 million and an estimated $12 million since it was founded in 2002. In the last seven years, *the Amish community has defaulted on only $1,300 in medical bills!*

I asked Ms. Siedler about her impressions of Amish as patients. She noted that they always want to know the cost of a procedure, such as a hip replacement, and postpone the surgery until they have the money to pay for it. When an Amish patient is discharged, the hospital gets paid with a check with no insurance forms to file. Typically a self-pay English person on discharge wants to set up a payment plan.

'When an Amish patient is discharged, the hospital gets paid with a check with no insurance forms to file.'

Recently an Amish man called Immergrun saying his wife needed gall bladder surgery. Ms. Siedler collected the medical record from the local doctor and sent it to a participating surgeon, then sent the patient the estimated cost of the procedure in nearby hospitals. The Amish woman contacted the surgeon who arranged for the surgery with the subsequent bills sent to Immergrun. In cases of an acute injury or illness, the Amish may have to go to a non-participating hospital where they will have to individually negotiate for their fees. Bishop H is clear that Immergrun has greatly facilitated the way that Amish pay their medical bills while respecting the Amish ways regarding their avoidance of insurance.

An Amish herbalist

As part of the research for this chapter, I went to see "Daniel," an Amish herbalist and naturopathic physician. I asked him how he got into herbal medicine.

Daniel said, "I have to tell you my story." For the next hour, Daniel told me the story of his own illness, which can be book in itself. At age 34 he was an accomplished plumber and thought this would be his life work. But he began to experience severe muscle and joint aching that didn't respond to treatment from his doctor. He was hospitalized with a diagnosis of meningitis and at one point was so sick that his family was called in to say their goodbyes.

Daniel was transferred to Mayo Clinic by airplane where he was again treated intensively for meningitis. His condition did not improve. His weight plummeted from 180 pounds to 134. With his strength nearly gone, his Mayo Clinic doctor came to see Daniel to discuss his condition. He said, "We are both human beings and we have a lot in common. But we have been brought up differently and see things differently. I am a doctor. You are a plumber. We need your help to figure out how the infection gets into your spinal fluid and causes the meningitis." Daniel understood from this conversation that the doctor was telling him that Mayo Clinic had nothing further to offer and that, if he was to survive, he needed to discover the cause himself. As they parted, the doctor said, "If you find out what the problem is, let us know."

Daniel went home by car from Minnesota to northern Indiana, his head on his wife's lap. After he arrived home, he picked up the nearest book on medical problems he could find and started reading. He tried some home remedies and, over a period of weeks, gained enough strength to work two days a week at a hardware store.

At the urging of a friend, Daniel entered a lengthy correspondence course in naturopathy. Over the next four years of this course, the lowest grade he got was a 97%. After completing the course, he entered a partnership with a chiropractor to sell natural products wholesale. With knowledge from his naturopathic studies, he began trying some of these products on himself and noticed improvement. He still didn't have a diagnosis for his symptoms. After several years, Daniel started a retail business selling natural remedies and in that role began to answer people's questions about natural products to take for various illnesses. Folks began to come to him for advice about their physical problems.

With his growing experience and clientele, Daniel started seeing clients by appointment. By this time he had extensive knowledge of naturally occurring products for a variety of ailments. Eventually, his son and another Amish young man completed the naturopathic training and joined him in seeing clients. Currently three naturopathic practitioners' schedules are filled with appointments by local people, as well as patients from as far away as Hawaii. Their clientele is about 60% Amish and 40% English.

> *When I had asked for an appointment with Daniel, the first available appointment was six weeks later. Daniel did have time over lunch the next day where I heard his remarkable story.*

I wanted to know more about how Daniel relates to the individuals who come to him. He responded readily and freely to my questions.

Q. Do you prescribe natural products?

We don't prescribe medicines. We *suggest* what people may do. I usually say something like, "If I were you, I would take this, or if you were someone in my family, I would suggest this remedy." When persons who are taking prescription medications from traditional doctors come to see me, I try to find a remedy for them from natural sources. When they ask what they should do about their present medicines, I tell them: "I didn't put you on the medicine, and I won't take you off that medicine."

Q. Are there circumstances when you refer your patients to traditional doctors?

Last week I had an Amish man all bent over in pain come to see me. He had come in by buggy and must have felt severe pain with every bounce of the buggy. His pain was in the right lower side of his abdomen, and his symptoms all suggested appendicitis. I told him he probably has appendicitis, arranged for a car and driver, and sent him to a doctor who transferred him to the local hospital for surgery.

Q. Do you save people money?

I don't charge people for my services. All the time I was sick, I prayed to God and felt that there was a purpose in all of that sickness. When I got better, I wanted to help people. [He earns income when people make purchases at his store that specializes in natural products.]

Several months ago a man with a stiff neck and headache came to see me. Based on my own experience, I knew it could be something serious like meningitis. I suggested a natural remedy, with strict orders that if he was not improving in three hours he should get in to see a traditional doctor. He called after three hours and said he felt improved. He called back again in two days and said he was feeling fine. The cost of his medicine was $16.95.

A woman from Pennsylvania who was mentally disturbed came to live with a family here in the area. She needed constant attention for her own protection; on one occasion she tried to throw herself in front of a truck. She had been on medication without improvement. I suggested that she take some natural remedies. The family reported that after a week she was less agitated, and four weeks later she appeared normal. If she had been hospitalized, the cost would have been in the thousands of dollars.

Q. Have you had any opposition from local doctors?

No, not from local doctors. Two times I had inquiries from officials with the state of Indiana. One was settled with my reply by letter to their inquiry and the other after discussion with three people who came to visit me here.

Q. Did you ever find out what was wrong with you during your long illness?

Yes, in 2005 I was playing around with a microscope and looked at a slide of my blood and saw some "squiggly" things. I am now convinced that I had Lyme disease. I could see that these squiggly things got less and less as I took some natural remedies.

Q. Did you ever tell the doctor at Mayo Clinic what you now believe was your sickness?

No, I don't remember his name, and it was so long ago.

Nurse/midwife

Kate Shantz is pleasant, middle-aged and smiles easily. She is a certified nurse/midwife with the required BSN and a master's degree in nursing with a focus on midwifery. She works alone and is on call 24 hours a day, seven days a week for her patients.

About 80% of her clients are Amish. More than half of her deliveries are in the homes of her Amish clients.

The Amish are very interested in the costs of their healthcare and usually ask up front what it will cost. When Amish clients call, Ms. Shantz describes her services, tells them the prices and makes sure they understand that she carries no malpractice insurance. No Amish family has objected.

Her professional charges include pre- and post-partum visits, delivery and initial well-baby care.
- Home delivery: $2,300
- Delivery in the birthing center: $1,500

Ms. Shantz feels that on occasion the Amish concern for the cost of care can become a problem in getting the best care. She recalls a pregnant woman who was in the process of a miscarriage and needed immediate attention. When informed that his wife needed to be in the hospital, her husband took out his sheet of paper with comparative prices at several hospitals. The Amish husband wanted to send his wife to a more distant hospital in order to save on costs. The woman needed immediate attention, and Ms. Shantz had to insist that they take her to the closest hospital, which they did.

'She recalls a pregnant Amish woman who was in the process of a miscarriage and needed immediate attention.'

Ms. Shantz enjoys working with the Amish. During the pre-natal course, pregnant women get advice from older women. They accept pregnancy and having babies as part of life. With this attitude, the delivery tends to be accepted as a normal part of life. Amish women generally prefer women to care for them and so prefer a midwife to a male doctor. Amish have no set rule about circumcising the male babies. After the delivery, an Amish maid comes to live in the home for at least several weeks. This may be a family relative or someone else from the community.

Conclusion

There are a number of factors in the ability of the Amish to cope with the high cost of healthcare.

- First, since they don't have insurance, it automatically places a greater emphasis on knowing the cost of care and thinking twice before elective surgery.
- Second, their innate self-sufficiency in all they do lends itself to finding local and home remedies for their illnesses.
- Third, they not only ask about prices but negotiate for lower prices.
- Fourth, the Amish have in some locations banded together to improve their ability to negotiate better prices.
- Fifth, the traditional system to assist one another in times of need is applied to paying for healthcare bills.

The three customary parameters of healthcare are access (the ability to get appropriate care when needed), quality (healthcare that meets the prevailing standard of care) and cost (usually defined as affordable). In general, the information presented here suggests that the Amish have found ways to get quality, affordable healthcare without outside insurance.

CHAPTER TWENTY-FIVE

Health and Wellness:
Doing What We *Know* to Do

In 1981 my wife and I started a community-based program in Bellefontaine, Ohio, that we called RENEW—an acronym for recreation, education, nutrition, exercise and wellness. We applied for and received a three-year grant for community-based, health-related programs from the U.S. Center for Disease Control[43] in competition with more than 250 other applicants. In 1981 wellness was a little-known concept.

Nearly 30 years ago we listed our objectives for a wellness program. These objectives are still applicable today:

- To promote the concept that health is more than the absence of the symptoms of disease and that we have unrealized potential to improve our quality of life and longevity.
- To help individuals indentify the lifestyle choices that will improve their health by modifying risk factors.
- To provide peer support through a group to make right choices.
- To encourage and coordinate the use of facilities and agencies within the community that will assist in changing lifestyles.
- To promote education of our children regarding the importance of good health habits, regular exercise and methods of coping with stress.
- To encourage educators to incorporate more life sports in the education of our children.

Groups of 25 people were organized and, at the opening session, introduced to the idea of wellness. We gave them a test that identified their risk factors. They then went through a six-week course with weekly sessions. In the first hour persons with expertise discussed diet, exercise, stress management, goal setting and personal responsibility. In the second hour, participants engaged in a supervised walking or jogging program. At the start, some of these people barely had the energy to walk around the quarter-mile track one time.

These groups quickly developed a spirit of helping each other to better health. Many people found others in the group with whom to walk between sessions, and some of the groups continued to meet after the six-week course was completed.

The good life

In our fantasies, the good life is free from worry, filled with pleasurable moments, good food, plenty of leisure time for relaxed lounging with stimulating and fun-loving friends, and enough money to do it all. In these fantasies, happiness and contentment fill our days.

But wait. When we look around it seems that the happiest people are not those with the most money and leisure time but rather people who have meaningful relationships. Their happiness has little to do with their external circumstances.

> *Rose, our housekeeper when we lived in Calcutta, told us of her life with an alcoholic husband and nine pregnancies in 12 years.[44] She was the main source of support for her family. Four of her children died of diseases that were preventable with normal immunizations and adequate healthcare. Yet Rose said of*

her family's seven years in the worst slums of Cal-
cutta, "We were so happy. We were poor, but so was
everyone else, and we all helped each other." Despite
her seemingly overwhelming difficulties, Rose was a
gracious host with a ready smile for everyone. Her
priorities were clear. One evening at the dinner table
she told us of her concern for her daughter and son-
in-law in London upon hearing they had just bought
a new car. Rose was uneasy that they "would have so
much that they couldn't help wanting more." Her per-
spective stands in marked contrast to multimillionaire
John D. Rockefeller who, upon being asked how much
money he wanted, reportedly replied with one word:
"More." Rose, on the other hand, embodied the con-
tented spirit of the Apostle Paul in the Book of Philip-
pians in the New Testament of the Bible.[45]

Rose's attitude is reflected among the people of Calcutta
whose expectations of what life owes them are low. For most
of them, it is enough to have assurance of adequate food to
place on the table, friends to share it with and a roof over
one's head. There is no sense of entitlement that defines what
one deserves. They are therefore spared the frustration of
high expectations not met.

'The good life is one filled with joy, an inner joy that has little to do with external circumstances.'

The good life is one filled with joy, an inner joy that has little
to do with external circumstances. That joy is a natural out-

come from a sense of gratitude. Gratefulness comes as we recall the good things in our lives. Most of the time when I dress myself, I have at least a fleeting thought about a friend with only one arm and wonder how she does the simple things like dressing herself. I am grateful for two arms.

Wellness

The key to wellness is to accept responsibility for one's own health. Essential to wellness is personal responsibility that says that I make many choices that have the possibility to do good or harm to my own health. It also recognizes that wellness enhances health beyond simply being free from disease or symptoms. A life committed to wellness recognizes that there are many things under my control that will contribute to more vigor and longer life.

A collaborative relationship with a primary healthcare provider can help achieve the goals of wellness. In this relationship, the doctor-provider says to the patient-consumer, "Your health is *your* responsibility. What you want, I want: to help you realize the best health possible to enable you live out your potential. I am here as a source of information and guidance for you to achieve that." The patient says to the doctor, "I know that my health is my responsibility. As we cooperate in this effort, I hope we can have an open and ongoing conversation about how to attain our common goal of maximizing my health."

But most of us tend to "put off the day" of making the necessary changes. Psychologists and educators say that just about everyone procrastinates. We delay what we know is important to do. Other things come up that seem equally important, or we think we need to keep "clearing the decks" before we undertake the important task.

Students find ways to delay starting to write term papers even though they know the assignment and the deadline. Others of us procrastinate in things like starting a proper diet, losing weight or building our saving accounts. I am convinced that when it comes to getting on with what we know to do in wellness, procrastination is the major culprit. So I decided to read about procrastination; I found good information by Googling[46] the subject.[47] I also discovered that I am not immune to this "disease" myself.

Procrastination

After I had read several accounts of procrastination, I was pretty sleepy, so I decided to take a nap so that my mind would be fresh to write about the subject. After I awoke, I got a cup of coffee to sharpen my thinking so I could express myself more clearly. To make sure that I had enough energy for my writing, I ate a small piece of cake.

When I got to my desk, I found some financial papers there and, in order to clear my work space so I could write more efficiently, I entered the numbers into the computer. While my mind was on finances, I thought I should check how the stock market was doing. While doing so, I noticed the *New York Times* headline about an earthquake in Italy and felt I needed to see if any famous monuments were damaged. And in the interest of efficiency, while I was online I checked my e-mail.

Then, in order to give me confidence before plunging into my writing, I felt I needed to succeed at something, so I decided to play a game of Free Cell on the computer. At that point, realizing I had just spent three hours procrastinating, I sat down to write about procrastination.

'Realizing I had just spent three hours procrastinating, I sat down to write about procrastination.'

This reflection in regard to procrastination is similar to the student who has to write a term paper. Notice that none of the things that I did to delay starting to write were bad things (well, maybe eating the cake). That's the way it is with procrastination. It's not that we're doing nothing, and most of what we're doing might be termed good things. But the end result is that I effectively delayed by three hours starting what I considered the most important—to write about procrastination.

As for wellness itself, there are many ways to become involved. The trick is, first, to simply start, then move from following the course of least resistance to taking charge of the different areas of life. Taking responsibility for oneself is the key to a life of wellness. Wellness measures can be as individual as eating right and regular exercise or community-wide, as the following account illustrates.

The U.S. Centers for Disease Control and Prevention reported on New Year's Day 2009 the result of a three-year study of three communities in Colorado on the effects of a smoking ban. There was a 41% reduction (257 to 152 per 100,000) in the incidence of heart attacks in the three years in Pueblo after a workplace smoking ban was enacted, compared with two neighboring communities with no smoking ban. This is the most extensive study that verifies the result of eight previous studies on the beneficial effects of communitywide smoking bans in the workplace.

Wellness is effective at any age

Further, a recent study[48] of 2,357 men over a 25-year period showed that modifying health-related risk factors at an older age can have a positive effect on both quality of life and longevity. At the start of the study, the average age of the men was 72. Detailed medical records were recorded. Forty-one percent lived past 90 years. The four identified factors that increased the probability of death were smoking, diabetes, obesity and high blood pressure. In the absence of any of these four conditions, the likelihood of living to 90-plus years of age was 54%. Elderly men who exercised regularly had nearly a 30% reduction in their risk of dying.

Men with healthy lifestyles who acquired a chronic illness were significantly older than those who had unhealthy lifestyles. Perhaps most significantly, the men with healthy lifestyles reported generally feeling better and were physically more vigorous. The study concluded that "Modifiable healthy behaviors during early elderly years, including smoking abstinence, weight management, blood pressure control, and regular exercise, are associated not only with enhanced life span in men but also with good health and function during older age."

Economic incentives for wellness and preventive medicine

Where does the incentive for preventive care come from— provider, consumer or business? It has been said that our healthcare system is not designed to promote health. It is rather to treat sickness. Yet intuitively we know that we can do much to promote good health through well-defined wellness programs.

Doctors have little incentive to promote wellness

The fee-for-service practice has been basic to our system of healthcare. For most primary practitioners this means that there will be limits in the time available for each patient. The average doctor in private practice has high office costs that are relatively fixed regardless of the number of patients that he or she sees. The electricity, building and employees must be paid.

Another pressure for the primary practitioner is the fact that the system of financial return favors procedures over the more mundane issues of everyday healthcare. Despite efforts by insurance companies and Medicare/Medicaid to address this problem, many primary care practitioners feel underpaid in comparison to their colleagues in practices with more procedures, such as colonoscopies, heart catheterizations or surgery.

Medical education is structured to emphasize the treatment of illness—to restore a presenting patient to a condition where such symptoms as pain, weakness or dizziness are gone. When that happens, the practitioner has done what the patient came for. Hopefully the doctor will discuss measures that can prevent the recurrence of the illness or symptoms. But the doctor is usually busy. In view of limited time and having met the main expectations of the patient, there is a tendency to give lip service to or slide lightly over education measures to prevent recurrences.

Business—and incentives for wellness measures

From 2000 to 2005 insurance costs went up 59% in the United States while wages increased by only 12%. Because of the escalating cost of insurance, business owners understandably must look for ways to decrease their healthcare costs. Small businesses increasingly find it difficult or impossible to provide health insurance for their employees. In the same five-year period the percentage of companies providing health insurance fell from 69% to 60%.

In an effort to decrease healthcare costs, some companies have instituted wellness measures for their employees. In order to motivate employees to better lifestyle habits, companies have used both the carrot and the stick methods: offer financial incentives to achieve wellness goals or penalize financially if goals are not met. The trend is toward the carrot method whereby the deductible co-pay will be reduced for employees who meet their wellness goals.

Do financial incentives work? In one large study, 878 employees were randomly assigned to two groups. One group was given educational materials on smoking cessation, while the second group was given the same information—plus financial incentives:
- $100 to complete the smoking cessation program
- $250 if they were not smoking at six months
- $400 if they were not smoking after another six months

The results showed a clear difference, with more than twice the number of persons who were offered the financial incentive quitting smoking.[49]

The evidence indicates that employers can lower their employee healthcare costs with wellness programs. The Center for Prevention and Health Services[50] quotes statistics that for every dollar spent on health promotion among employees there was a saving of $3.48 on employee medical expenses and a saving of $5.82 on the cost of absenteeism. This represents about a 9 to 1 return on the dollars spent in healthcare wellness programs by business.

Consumers' financial incentives for wellness

We have considered the financial incentives for doctors and businesses to promote prevention and wellness. How about the consumer?

Multiple studies confirm that people with obesity, diabetes, alcoholism and nicotine addiction have significantly higher healthcare costs and reduced life expectancy than others without these conditions. In addition to the direct healthcare costs, there is the added immense cost of absenteeism from work and early disability.

Conclusion

In addition to the prospect for a longer life, making good lifestyle choices will result in a new image, better self-esteem, more appetite for living, and a longer and more fulfilled life. The lower costs also will put money in your pocket that otherwise would have been spent on maintaining your health.

'Making good lifestyle choices
will result in a new image,
better self-esteem, more appetite
for living, and a longer
and more fulfilled life.'

Several factors may change the economic incentives for preventive healthcare. If there's a mass move toward a single-payer system to finance healthcare, it will be to everyone's benefit that more illnesses are prevented and better care for chronic disease is available. In a single-payer method, the financial risk is shared by all. Now most insurance companies generally seek to insure only the healthiest among us. Persons with a pre-existing illness are either refused insurance or pay exorbitant, even prohibitive, fees.

Many of these conditions are entirely preventable and within the control of the individual. The evidence is clear: Good lifestyle choices are effective and will improve the quality of life—and reduce the cost of healthcare. The choice is mine—and yours—to make. In the words of Deuteronomy 30:19:

> *Today I have given you the choice between life and death, between blessings and curses. Now I call on heaven and earth to witness the choice you make. Oh, that you would choose life, so that you and your descendants might live!* (New Living Translation *of the Bible*)

ENDNOTES

Introduction

[1] "Financing Health Care Reform," Editorial, *New York Times,* July 6, 2009.

[2] Atul Gawande, "The Cost Conundrum: What a Texas Town Can Teach Us About Health Care," *The New Yorker,* June 1, 2009.

[3] L. Yasaitis, E. S. Fisher, J. S. Skinner & A. Chandra. "Hospital Quality and Intensity of Spending: Is There an Association?" Dartmouth Institute for Health Policy and Clinical Practice, Hanover, NH 03755, *Journal of Ambulatory Care Management,* July–September 2009, Vol. 32, No. 3, pages 226–231.

Chapter 2

[4] David M. Studdert, William M. Sage, et al., "Defensive Medicine Widespread, with Serious Consequences," *Journal of the American Medical Association* (JAMA), June 1, 2005.

[5] Ibid.

Chapter 4

[6] While the Internet is the source of an immense amount of information, a word of caution is in order. Not all of this information is true. Scammers, frauds and pornographers can—and do—post on the Internet. So do people with medical information and cures that are inaccurate and unfounded. Check the accuracy of any information with a reliable source, such as Merck Manual at *http://www.merck.com/mmpe/index.html.*

Chapter 10

[7] The National Center for Complementary and Alternative Medicine defines complementary and alternative medicine (CAM) as: "A group of diverse medical and health care systems, practices, and products that are not presently considered to be part of conventional medicine." The website had an extensive classification of CAM. The list of practices that are considered CAM changes continually, as those therapies that are proven to be safe and effective become adopted into conventional healthcare and as new approaches to healthcare emerge.
http://nccam.nih.gov/health/whatiscam/. Accessed June 20, 2009.

Chapter 16

[8] *Calcutta Telegraph*, December 10, 1992.

[9] In the spirit of Matthew 5:48 where Jesus says in the Sermon on the Mount: "Be perfect, therefore, as your heavenly Father is perfect" (*New International Version* of the Bible).

Chapter 18

[10] Jennifer E. DeVoe, M.D., D.Phil.; Lorraine S. Wallace, Ph.D.; Nancy Pandhi, M.D., M.P.H.; Rachel Solotaroff, M.D.; & George E. Fryer Jr., Ph.D., "Comprehending Care in a Medical Home: A Usual Source of Care and Patient Perceptions About Healthcare Communication," *Journal of the American Board of Family Medicine,* 2008, Vol. 21, No. 5, pages 441–450. © 2008 American Board of Family Medicine.

Chapter 19

[11] "The Altered Human Is Already Here," *New York Times,* April 2, 2004.

[12] See *http://www.sourcewatch.org/index.php?title=Direct-to-consumer advertising.* Accessed May 4, 2009.

[13] *Agency for Healthcare Research and Quality (AHRQ) Publication Number 01-0020,* "Reducing and Preventing Adverse Drug Events to Decrease Hospital Costs," *http://www.ahrq.gov/qual/aderia/aderia.html.* Accessed March 26, 2009.

[14] "Cancer Facts and Figures 2005," American Cancer Society, Atlanta, Georgia, 2005.

Chapter 21

[15] "Dying in an Acute Hospital Setting: The Challenges and Solutions," Rasha Al-Qurainy, M.D., Emily Collis, M.D., David Feuer, M.D., *International Journal of Clinical Practice,* 2009, Vol. 63, No. 3, pages 508–515. © 2009 Blackwell Publishing.

[16] See *http://www.euthanasia.com/index.html.* Accessed July 7, 2009.

Chapter 22

[17] David M. Ellsberg, M.D., et al., "Trends in Alternative Medicine in the United States, 1990–1997," *Journal of the American Medical Association* (JAMA), 1998, Vol. 280, pages 1569–1575.

[18] In the early 20th century, medical education was unregulated and consisted of a loose apprenticeship with an established doctor. "Medical Schools" were operated to turn a profit. All this changed after the Flexner Report. Abraham Flexner researched and wrote a report on the state of medical education in United States and Canada. His report, written in 1910, eventually led to reform and standardization of medical education.

[19] R. Alton Lee, *The Bizarre Careers of John R. Brinkley,* University Press of Kentucky, 2002.

[20] "Complementary Medicine: Time for Critical Engagement," *Lancet,* December 16, 2003, Vol. 356, No. 9247, page 2023.

[21] Hans Kocher, "Digitalis purpurea," Medical Botany Department of Biology, Texas A&M University, 1997, *http://www.csdl. tamu.edu/FLORA/Wilson/481/medbot/bot2.html*. Accessed August 24, 2005.

[22] William Withering (1741–99), a British physician, was known to his community for giving free service to needy patients. However, he is best known for introducing digitalis into medical practice.

Chapter 23

[23] "Infant Mortality and Life Expectancy for Selected Countries, 2007," *http://www.infoplease.com/ipa/A0004393.html*. Accessed February 2, 2009.

[24] Steffie Woolhander, M.D., M.P.H., Terry Campbell, M.H.A., and David U. Hummelstein, M.D. "Costs of Health Care Administration in the United States and Canada," *New England Journal of Medicine,* August 21, 2003, Vol. 349, pages 768–775.

[25] Uwe E. Reinhardt, "How Do Hospitals Get Paid? A Primer," *http://content.healthaffairs.org/cgi/content/abstract/25/1/57.* Accessed February 4, 2009.

[26] Shannon Brownlee, "Why Does Healthcare Cost So Much?" American Association of Retired Persons (AARP), July/August 2008.

[27] See the American College of Radiology (ARC) website at *http://www.qualityimaging.org/index.asp*. Accessed February 4, 2009.

[28] M. J. Frederich, "Neuroscience Becomes Image Conscious as Brain Scans Raise Ethical Issues," *Journal of the American Medical Association* (JAMA), 2005, Vol. 294, pages 781–783.

[29] Janet K. Freberger, et al., "The Rising Incidence of Chronic Low Back Pain," *Archives of Internal Medicine,* February 9, 2009, Vol. 169, No. 3, pages 251–258.

[30] "Too Many Doctors in the House," Op-Ed by David C. Goodman, *New York Times,* July 10, 2006.

[31] Berkeley Rice, "Malpractice Rates: How High Now?" *Medical Economics,* January 9, 2004.

Chapter 24

[32] Most of the research for this chapter was done among the Amish in northern Indiana—one of the three large Amish communities in North America. The other two are in southeastern Pennsylvania and east-central Ohio. It should be noted that the Amish in other communities have variations on the methods of paying for healthcare described here.

[33] An Amish friend describes the process of choosing a minister by lot. The bishop, assisted by another bishop, sits by an open window of the house where the meeting is held. All members of the congregation pass by and state their choice for minister. Five men receive a set number of votes and are considered candidates. During the following week, the two bishops visit each of the candidates and their wives and ask them if they are willing to serve if selected. On the next Sunday, the bishop in charge places on a table before the congregation identical hymnbooks equal to the number of candidates. In each hymnbook the bishop has placed a thin slip of paper. One slip had the words from Proverbs 16:33: "The lot is cast into the lap; but its every decision is of the Lord" (*New International Version* of the Bible). The bishop then offers a prayer for divine guidance. Each candidate chooses one of the books. The bishop opens the books in turn until he finds the lot slip. The candidate in whose book the lot slip was found is then affirmed as chosen by God to be the minister. The chosen one is immediately ordained.

[34] If a family is in trouble with creditors, three men are appointed to take over the family checkbook, place the family on a strict budget and gradually pay off the creditors.

[35] See *Amish Grace: How Forgiveness Transcended Tragedy* by Donald B. Kraybill, Steven M. Nolt and David L. Weaver-Zercher, pages 163–167. This book gives an account of the West Nickel Mines School tragedy where five young Amish girls were killed and five more critically injured by a distraught Charles Carl Roberts IV. The book recounts the immediate and remarkable forgiveness expressed by the Amish community after the shooting.

[36] A re-enactment of a barn raising is prominent in "Witness," a 1985 U.S. film directed by Peter Weir and starring Harrison Ford. This movie is one of the most accurate and sensitive popular depictions of Amish life and culture.

[37] Samuel L. Yoder, "Brauche." *Global Anabaptist Mennonite Encyclopedia Online.* 1989. Global Anabaptist Mennonite Encyclopedia Online, *http://www.gameo.org/encyclopedia/contents/B7398ME.html*. Accessed April 29, 2009.

[38] S. S. Stoltzfus, "Plain Talk on Health Care: What's Your Opinion?" Special to the *Sunday News* (Lancaster, Pennsylvania), In My Opinion, August 10, 2008, Section P, page P1.

[39] J. Winfield Fretz, Harold S. Bender and Laban Peachey. "Mutual Aid." *Global Anabaptist Mennonite Encyclopedia Online,* 1989, Global Anabaptist Mennonite Encyclopedia Online, *http://www.gameo.org/encyclopedia/contents/M88ME*. Accessed June 9, 2009.

[40] The principal passages from the Bible that have been used to support the practice of shunning are Matthew 18:15–17, Romans 16:17, I Corinthians 5:11–13, II Thessalonians 3:6,14–15 and II John 10–11. The interpretation of these passages has varied among Christian groups over the centuries.

[41] By comparison, the administrative cost is 20–31% for commercial insurance and 4.9% for Medicare/Medicaid. The administrative cost is lower for Immergrun than commercial insurance because with direct cash payment to the hospital on discharge, there is no need for people to shuffle through the insurance claims. In addition, compared with commercial insurance, Immergrun doesn't have employees devising new product lines, no sales people, no advertising and doesn't need to make a profit. Immergrun's expenses include the salaries of two and a half employees, travel expense, and office overhead for electricity and $600 per month rent.

[42] Cindy Siedler pays each bill as it arrives and bills the Amish family on a monthly basis. She carefully checks the bills for duplicate charges or charges for services not given.

Chapter 25

[43] The name has since been changed to U.S. Centers for Disease Control and Prevention.

[44] *Rose: A Story of Faith and Courage in Calcutta,* by Glen E. Miller, M.D. Available at *http://secure.mcc.org/mccstore/index.php?main_page=advanced _search_result&search_in_description=1&keyword=Rose&subm it.x=8&submit.y=5&submit=Search.*

[45] "I am not saying this because I am in need, for I have learned to be content whatever the circumstances. I know what it is to be in need, and I know what it is to have plenty. I have learned the secret of being content in every situation, whether well fed or hungry, whether living in plenty or in want. I can do everything through [God] who gives me strength" (Philippians 4:11–13, *New International Version* of the Bible).

46 Student Academic Services, California Polytechnic State University, *http://sas.calpoly.edu/asc/ssl/procrastination.html.* Accessed April 6, 2009.

47 "Hidden Reasons Students Procrastinate: Based on Procrastination Studies,"
http://video.google.com/videosearch?q=procrastination&sourcei d=navclient-ff&rlz=1B3RNFA_enUS267US268&um=1&ie= UTF-8&ei=TmHaScK1KqnulQeKyZThDA&sa=X&oi= video_result_group&resnum=4&ct=title#. Accessed April 6, 2009.

48 Laurie Barclay, M.D., "Modifiable Healthy Behaviors May Improve Life Span, Health, Function in Older Men," *Archives of Internal Medicine,* February 11, 2009.

49 Kevin G. Volpp, et al., "A Randomized, Controlled Trial of Financial Incentives for Smoking Cessation ...," *New England Journal of Medicine,* February 12, 2009, Vol. 360, No. 7, pages 699–709.

50 Part of the U.S. Centers for Disease Control and Prevention.

ACKNOWLEDGMENTS

There are many, many people who contributed to this book—from its inception to the final version you hold in your hands.

Dan Shenk of CopyProof, my editor, leads the list of individuals deserving my thanks for his professional expertise, advice and encouragement. The working relationship with him made the editing process enjoyable, with free give and take on how to best turn a phrase or communicate an idea. He also suggested several subject areas for inclusion that made the book more complete.

Two focus groups helped shape the responses to the doctor-patient encounters. I appreciate Kathy Brewton's leadership of the focus group at Greencroft Retirement Center and Greencroft's decision to allow 10 employees to meet with me regularly over a period of eight weeks. Thanks also to the focus group comprising four doctors, three nurse practitioners, several hospital nurses, and a hospital chaplain for their energy and thoughtful input.

My family gave both encouragement and expertise. Thanks to Marilyn, my wife, for her support and patience as I disappeared into my office for hours at a time, and to my daughter Korla and son Ed who gave valuable and insightful input, particularly in the way the message of the doctor-patient encounters could best be communicated. In writing this book, I have realized the value of having two children with English majors in the family!

I also want to thank the many people who read parts of the manuscript and gave helpful suggestions and encouragement, along with faithful friends who regularly sent me pertinent news articles that helped me keep up with the fast-moving healthcare discussions of recent months and years.

ABOUT THE AUTHOR

Glen Miller was born in northwestern Ohio into a family of nine children. He can trace his heritage back through 13 generations of Mennonites. At an early age he decided to become a doctor, motivated by the story of a young physician who left the glitter of a large city, giving up wealth, to serve the mountain people of eastern Kentucky. Glen, who had no money for higher education, was able to get his pre-medical education by working nights while going to school during the day. He is a 1957 graduate of Goshen (Indiana) College and 1961 graduate of Western Reserve University School of Medicine, Cleveland, Ohio.

For 25 years Dr. Miller worked as a primary care physician and hospital administrator in Bellefontaine, Ohio. With his wife, Marilyn, he lived overseas in Haiti and Egypt, where he worked as a doctor and medical teacher. Later they lived and worked in India for seven years, in Cambodia as interim directors of a development program and for nine months in London as hosts at a peace center.

Dr. Miller's seven years in India as the director of a large community development program provided insights that contributed to the writing of *Empowering the Patient*. In his association with the development program, he became a strong proponent of empowerment—the process of building the capacity of powerless people to influence events in their favor. Through education and organization, Dr. Miller saw people catch a vision of engagement and empowerment that changed their lives. The intent behind *Empowering the Patient* is that readers will catch a similar vision.

Glen and Marilyn have four children and nine grandchildren. Among their children and spouses are educators, social workers, a physician, a nurse and a healthcare researcher. The Millers make their home in Goshen, Indiana.

LaVergne, TN USA
06 December 2009
166154LV00002B/140/P